"A fantastic guidebook for people with back or neck pain."
—Dean Edell, M.D., author of *Eat, Drink, and Be Merry*

Renowned physical therapist Robin McKenzie shares his innovative program, which has become the first treatment of choice for back and neck care in 35 countries, including the United States. In *7 Steps to a Pain-Free Life*, you'll read about:

- Common causes of lower-back and neck pain
- The vital role discs play in back and neck health
- The simple exercises that alleviate pain immediately
- How to stay out of pain

Plus:

- Common back remedies and solutions
- How to alleviate acute lower-back pain
- How to alleviate acute neck pain
- Illuminating case studies—and real solutions

"I think Robin McKenzie's work is wonderful."
—Art Brownstein, M.D., author of *Healing Back Pain Naturally*

"The McKenzie Method has become a keystone for back and neck care, and this book is an invaluable tool for better health."
—HealthNewsDigest.com

ROBIN MCKENZIE is a world-renowned physical therapist who has spent the last forty years perfecting the McKenzie Method, hailed as the ultimate cure for back and neck pain. In 1990, he was named Officer of the Most Excellent Order of the British Empire (OBE) by Queen Elizabeth II. In January 2000, he was appointed to Companion of the New Zealand Order of Merit (CNZM). Mr. McKenzie lives in New Zealand.

CRAIG KUBEY is the author of seven previous books. He lives in California.

Also by Robin McKenzie

Treat Your Own Back

Treat Your Own Neck

The Cervical and Thoracic Spine: Mechanical Diagnosis and Therapy

The Lumbar Spine: Mechanical Diagnosis and Therapy

The Human Extremities: Mechanical Diagnosis and Therapy

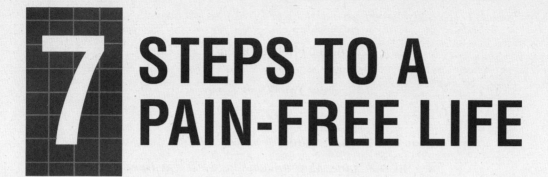

7 STEPS TO A PAIN-FREE LIFE

HOW TO RAPIDLY RELIEVE BACK AND NECK PAIN

Robin McKenzie with Craig Kubey

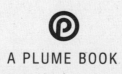

A PLUME BOOK

PUBLISHER'S NOTE

Every effort has been made to ensure that the information contained in this book is complete and accurate. However, neither the author nor the publisher is engaged in rendering professional advice or services to the individual reader. The ideas, procedures, and suggestions contained in this book are not intended as a substitute for consulting with your physician. All matters regarding your health require medical supervision. Neither the author nor the publisher shall be liable or responsible for any loss, injury, or damage allegedly arising from any information or suggestion in this book.

PLUME
Published by the Penguin Group
Penguin Putnam Inc., 375 Hudson Street, New York, New York 10014, U.S.A.
Penguin Books Ltd, 27 Wrights Lane, London W8 5TZ, England
Penguin Books Australia Ltd, Ringwood, Victoria, Australia
Penguin Books Canada Ltd, 10 Alcorn Avenue, Toronto, Ontario, Canada M4V 3B2
Penguin Books (N.Z.) Ltd, 182–190 Wairau Road, Auckland 10, New Zealand

Penguin Books Ltd, Registered Offices: Harmondsworth, Middlesex, England

Published by Plume, a member of Penguin Putnam Inc.
Previously published in a Dutton edition.

First Plume Printing, October 2001
2 4 6 8 6 10 9 7 5 3 1

REGISTERED TRADEMARK—MARCA REGISTRADA

The Library of Congress has catalogued the Dutton edition as follows:
LIBRARY OF CONGRESS CATALOGING-IN-PUBLICATION DATA
McKenzie, Robin.
7 Steps to a pain-free life: how to rapidly relieve back and neck pain
using the McKenzie method / Robin McKenzie with Craig Kubey.
p.   cm.
ISBN 0-525-94560-1 (hc.)
ISBN 0-452-28277-2 (pbk.)
1. Backache—Alternative treatment.   2. Neck pain—Alternative treatment.   3. Backache–
Exercise therapy.   4. Neck pain—Exercise therapy.   5. Self-care, Health.   I. Title: Seven
steps to a pain-free life.   II. Kubey, Craig   III. Title.

RD771.B217 M436 2000
617.5'6406—dc21
00-033567

Printed in the United States of America

BOOKS ARE AVAILABLE AT QUANTITY DISCOUNTS WHEN USED TO PROMOTE PRODUCTS OR SERVICES.
FOR INFORMATION PLEASE WRITE TO PREMIUM MARKETING DIVISION, PENGUIN PUTNAM INC.,
375 HUDSON STREET, NEW YORK, NEW YORK 10014.

To my wife
Joy

Contents

Acknowledgments

Robin McKenzie

To my patients who entrusted me with their care over the past forty years, I give my thanks and gratitude for teaching me all I know. I pass this on to you, the reader, and trust that you too can benefit.

Craig Kubey

I am grateful to the many McKenzie-affiliated health practitioners in the U.S. who generously provided advice and other assistance in connection with this book. They include Vert Mooney, M.D., Ron Donelson, M.D., and McKenzie-credentialed physical therapists Dave Pleva, Todd Edelson, Gudrun Morgan, Aidan O'Connor, Mary Sheid, Gerald Stern, Mary Stern, and Mark Werneke. Thanks also to Stacey Lyon of the McKenzie Institute U.S.A., who helped to put me in touch with the preceding physical therapists. I also thank Alan Kubey for computer assistance and Karen Kubey for photography; I thank them as well as Maki Kubey and Elizabeth Kubey for putting up with my work on this book.

Both of us

We thank our literary agency, RLR Associates (Jonathan Diamond, Lisa Dicker, Jennifer Unter, Manuela Barbuiani, Gretchen Topping, Jason White, et al.), for its diligent work on this project. Further, we express our appreciation to the editorial, production, and publicity people at Dutton (beginning with editor in chief Brian Tart; his assistant, Kara Howland; and copyeditor John Paine) for their extensive efforts to meet the extraordinary demands of the project that produced this book. Finally, we thank Jan McKenzie, general manager of Spinal Publications New Zealand Ltd., who handled the New Zealand administrative side of this project with extraordinary intellect, effort, diligence, diplomacy, and humor.

Dedications

Robin McKenzie's dedication appears on page v. Craig Kubey dedicates this book to his wife, Maki.

Introduction

by Craig Kubey

Introductions to important books are usually written by experts or celebrities. Or, even better, by experts who *are* celebrities. But I am neither an expert nor a celebrity. I am an attorney who gave up a public service legal career to become a writer. But most important to you, the reader, I am a beneficiary of the McKenzie Method. And I want you to be a beneficiary too.

As you read these words, it is likely (because you chose to pick up this book) that you have back pain or neck pain. I've been there. The main reason I'm not there right now is Robin McKenzie.

I have had plenty of good luck in my life and plenty of bad, but I have had the astonishingly bad luck to have had not just one whiplash injury caused by a rear-end auto collision, but three. I have also had the more common experience of developing lower back pain during my forties.

Because there are more back patients than neck patients, let's start with the back. For years I had occasional minor, very tolerable lower back pain for no reason known to me. But I'm a runner: track and cross-country in high school, track at the University of California, Berkeley. One day on a family trip to Santa Cruz, California, I went for a short run in some rolling hills. No back pain during the run.

But when I stopped, I had back pain that was *severe*. My family was a mile away, and it was a painful struggle to walk back to them. Back home, the pain was even worse. I remember one day when my wife and I were downtown and the car was half a block away. I asked her to go to the car and pick me up: the back pain was bad enough that I didn't even want to walk that half block.

But having already benefitted from the McKenzie exercises for the neck, I read the McKenzie exercises for the back. I focused on Exercise 3, Extension in Lying. Immediately, the back pain was better. In a few days it was so minor that it was of no concern to me.

I also learned that I was wrong in my analysis of what had happened. People who run without pain but find their backs hurting immediately afterward blame the running. Same thing with other sports. But McKenzie says—and my experience has borne this out—that typically the problem is not the exercise but what one does afterward. My run had been short, but it had been in hills and had been at a fairly rapid pace. So when I finished, I was out of breath, and I bent over, hands on knees, just as so many runners and other athletes do after so many types of exercise. This is where I made my mistake. Every indication is that if I had maintained a good posture right after the run, the back symptoms never would have arisen.

Now to all those whiplash injuries. The first one occurred in 1976. I was stopped at a stop sign and my car was struck by a big Cadillac. I was a member of an early health maintenance organization, and right after my injury, there was no way that HMO would let me see an orthopedist. I saw my family doctor there, but after several weeks my symptoms hadn't gotten much better. So without asking for a referral, I made an appointment with an orthopedist. He had eight patients an hour, and he spent most of our short time together expressing his astonishment that I had gotten to see him at all.

In search of relief, I eventually saw seven doctors: one primary care physician and six orthopedists. I was treated with heat, ultrasound, hands-on physical therapy, aspirin (this was before ibuprofen), Valium (as a muscle relaxant), and a hard cervical collar followed by a soft cervical collar. All of these things helped some, but none helped in any dramatic way. The pain persisted for more than a year and interfered seriously with my work and social life. I think the only thing that really got rid of the persistent neck pain was the passage of time—September 1976 to January 1978. The only McKenzie I knew about then was a guy in my high school class who played the drums in a rock band.

The next rear-end auto collision came in May 1986. While I was waiting to turn left at an intersection, my car was struck by a Ford Taurus. I was in a lot of pain once again. But this time I went to just one primary care physician and one orthopedist, who referred me to a physical therapist. For months this physical therapist and his associate treated me with hands-on therapies. These two seemed to know their business much better than the physical therapist of 1976, and almost every time I left their office, I felt much better, but for only about a day.

But eventually this physical therapist introduced me to the McKenzie exercises. I gave them a try once in a while, maybe one session on one day (you're supposed to do them about every two hours), then again some weeks later (you're supposed to do them every day until your symptoms get better). They provided a little relief, but the physical therapist didn't impress upon me the full value of these exercises or the importance of doing them *religiously*, which is to say to do them exactly as McKenzie would have you do them, and to stick with them. Nor did he seem to recognize that certain McKenzie exercises are tailored to certain situations (such as one-sided pain, which is what I had). So my treatment remained mostly of the hands-on variety. And the symptoms again took more than a year to fully resolve.

In 1993, I had a serious flare-up of my neck condition. This was caused when, as I parked my car, I ran into a curb at moderate speed. Most people would not have been bothered by this, but because of my previous neck injuries, within 15 minutes I had sharp pain.

But almost right away I remembered the McKenzie exercises, Exercise 1 (Head Retraction in Sitting) in particular. I did this exercise one time. That is, I retracted my head one time and held the position for about three seconds. The neck pain vanished all at once! In three seconds! (Years later I talked with a McKenzie-trained chiropractor, who said, "That's great when that happens, isn't it?" He had seen these instant cures with many patients.)

I'm not saying the McKenzie Method is ordinarily so successful that you can spend three seconds with it and be pain-free. Chances are small you will be that lucky. But once in a while it's just that powerful. And often the first session of exercises provides relief that, while not complete, is quite noticeable.

Auto collision whiplash number three happened in 1995: a Nissan pickup truck. The pain this time was not generally as severe as in the two other accidents, but it just hung on and hung on through several doctors and one physical therapist. I tried the McKenzie head-retraction exercise a few times, and it helped some, but not enough. The pain went on for more than a year.

Maybe I should have learned my lesson earlier, but I did not learn it until *after* the resolution of this third whiplash.

That 1995 auto accident was the last one. But there were countless flare-ups, generally associated with driving. In particular, if I'd strike a curb while parking, I'd have immediate pain. It usually would persist for about a day.

After one such micro-collision, the pain was sharper than usual, and it was on one side. I decided to review the McKenzie exercises more carefully. I skimmed through Exercises 1–4 and then came to Exercise 5 (Side-bending of the Neck). I realized for the first time that this exercise was for the specific situation I was in: pain mostly or exclusively on one side. My pain was on the right side, probably because the pain from the 1995 accident had been there. It had gone away but had left me vulnerable.

I did Exercise 5 a few times, and the pain was dramatically reduced in the very first session. I did it for one or two more sessions the same day, and it was just about gone. Soon it had entirely disappeared.

So my message is this: *don't skim, don't be careless, don't just glance at the exercises and make a "reasonable" attempt.* There is *genius* in these exercises, but you must do them *exactly* as Robin McKenzie says. Read every word of every exercise and figure out which one or ones fit your back pain or your neck pain. Do the exercise or exercises *exactly* as Robin instructs you. Do it as many times as he says in each session. Do it as many times a day as he says to, if your schedule in any way permits that. And do the exercises in the right order. If Robin says to do Exercise 1, then 6, then 1, and then 2, do them in that order! This guy McKenzie has been developing these exercises since 1956, and he knows what he's talking about.

You will know all this in your heart only once you have followed his advice (and mine here). When you find out just how right he is, it's an emotional experience. When the pain suddenly declines or even vanishes, you feel relieved, you feel grateful. You feel like finding out how to reach McKenzie and calling him on the phone. His wisdom is seen not just in the results you get, but in your experience as you do the exercises.

Exercise 2 (Neck Extension in Sitting) is a great example of this. Robin says to retract your head, then tilt it back as though looking at the sky, then, with your head tilted, repeatedly turn your nose a half-inch from the midline to the right and left, all the while tilting still farther back. It's amazing to find that even though you thought you had tilted your head back all the way, you can tilt it still farther back—but only if you turn your nose a little to the right, then to the left, just as he says.

I have paid the price for not following the McKenzie exercises closely enough. No one—no doctor, no physical therapist—had told me how important it was to do the exercises exactly as Robin McKenzie would have you do them. I've paid the price in years of pain and hundreds of medical and physical therapy appointments, 95 percent of which I now believe were unnecessary and therefore a waste of valuable time, not to mention my insurance company's money and my own (those co-payments).

Despite my emphasis on the exercises, it's important to stress two other facts. One is that although McKenzie is known for "extension"—bending the back or neck to a straight position or past that position—his method is much more than that. Even his exercises in some cases involve flexion, which is the opposite of extension. The other is that a back or neck patient will do best if he or she focuses on more than the exercises. That is, the reader should understand the entire McKenzie Method, which includes not only the exercises but a brief discussion of human anatomy, and which concentrates heavily on correct posture as both a preventive and corrective means of dealing with back and neck pain.

Two additional personal points:

1. When you have back or neck pain, especially neck pain, you may feel that your painful area is too fragile to mess around with. Your instinct may be to use ice, lie down, not risk making the injury worse. If you have a legitimate medical concern here, such as a serious injury, sure, rest, see a doctor, be sure it's safe to do the exercises. If it's your first neck injury, Robin himself says to see a doctor before using the exercises.

But if your injury isn't severe, just painful, try the exercises. You may be amazed to find that you probably aren't so fragile after all. You can tolerate the exercises. You may feel very rapid relief.

2. If you don't feel immediate relief, remember what McKenzie will tell you: sometimes relief doesn't come right away, sometimes the exercises are painful and you are no better after a session or two or a day or two. But stick with them. You will in all likelihood benefit from your patience.

They say converts are the most impassioned believers, and I've been converted from hoping doctors and physical therapists can help me to realizing that with McKenzie's exercises I can help myself. When I have a back or neck injury or a flare-up, no longer do I wait helplessly for someone to schedule me for an appointment: I read the McKenzie exercises and follow them to the letter. You can too. You should too.

Learn the McKenzie Method, learn the exercises, then do them exactly as instructed. You will very likely be completely free of pain in a surprisingly short amount of time. From one back/neck sufferer to another, I want you to know that this book may be the most effective doctor you have ever had.

—CRAIG KUBEY

7 STEPS TO A
PAIN-FREE LIFE

Preface:
The Chance Discovery

I practice physiotherapy in New Zealand. In the different English spoken in the United States, this means I am a physical therapist. In 1956, I was only a few years into my career when a "Mr. Smith" came into the office. He complained of pain that extended from the right side of his lower back to his right knee. It was difficult for him to stand upright. He could bend forward, but he could not bend backward. For three weeks I treated him with heat and ultrasound. These were well-accepted therapeutic techniques then and remain so now. Nevertheless, Mr. Smith did not improve at all.

Then, late on a Wednesday, Mr. Smith came in for another appointment. I greeted him and said, "Go into that treatment room, please. Undress and then lie facedown on the table, and I'll be in to see you."

Mr. Smith complied—to the letter. I didn't know it, but another physiotherapist had left the therapy table at an odd angle: the front was elevated 45 degrees. Mr. Smith lay facedown on that table, his pelvis and legs horizontal, his torso sharply elevated in a position called *extension*.

But I got a phone call, and then another physiotherapist needed to consult me. And so five minutes passed before I could attend to Mr. Smith. I knocked on his door, walked briskly in, and then froze. To my horror, I saw Mr. Smith lying in the bizarre position just described. Not only was the position odd; in 1956 the position was considered by the medical profession to be one that would cause damage to most any patient. I thought, "My God! What has he done? Has he made his injury much worse?"

"How are you doing, Mr. Smith?" I asked gingerly.

"It's the best I've been," he replied in sunny tones. "All the pain in the leg is gone."

I was astounded and mightily relieved, but I wanted to know more. "How's the low back?" I inquired.

"The funny thing is, the pain is a little worse, but it's moved from the right side over to the center."

"How are you tolerating that pain?"

"Better. It's better when it's in the middle there."

Then he stood up.

He could do this without pain!

I asked him to try carefully to bend forward and backward. As you will recall, previously he could bend forward but not backward.

Now, after those five minutes in that strange position, he suddenly could bend backward with only minor pain.

His standing up did nothing to reverse the gains he had experienced on the table: there still was no pain in his leg, and the back pain remained centralized.

I began to recover my equilibrium. "Oh yes, that's fine," I said, stumbling only a little. But I wanted to be sure no damage had been done. "Could you walk around a bit?" I asked him.

Mr. Smith walked around the treatment room. He walked quite normally. I was relieved. I felt that he had improved so much that we could ask for nothing more that day.

"Well, that's long enough for today," I said. "Come back tomorrow and we'll try it again."

The next day, Mr. Smith was back. And we repeated the same "treatment." After Mr. Smith had maintained that odd position on the table for about five minutes, all of his remaining symptoms were gone.

Mr. Smith taught me about extension. Learning from his remarkable recovery, I was able to develop exercises and postural-correction techniques involving extension and, later, flexion. On the following pages I will explain all of these to you. Thanks to Mr. Smith, you are probably just one book away from being well on the road to recovery.

IMPORTANT: If you have severe back or neck pain or are having your first episode of back or neck pain, do not use this book. See a physician or other health-care provider.

If you are now suffering from acute lower back pain, and have previously consulted a health-care provider about your back pain, skip to Chapter 7, "Instructions for People with Acute Lower Back Pain."

Similarly, if you have acute neck pain *right now*, and have previously consulted a health-care provider about your neck pain, skip to Chapter 14, "Instructions for People with Acute Neck Pain."

If you have back or neck pain that troubles you but is not acute, start with Chapter 1.

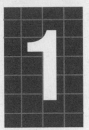

You Can Stop Back and Neck Pain

I don't claim to have spent years of research attempting to find a new and more effective means for treating back and neck pain. In a flash, those means found me. At least I had the presence of mind to recognize a powerful new therapy when it presented itself. And so, through the willingness of Mr. Smith to follow his physiotherapist's advice no matter how ridiculous, I discovered the power of extension. My colleagues and I now refer to the experience with Mr. Smith as "The Chance Discovery." With Mr. Smith and other patients, I rapidly realized that extension is often the key to prompt and effective self-treatment of back pain.

Over the span of four decades, I have continuously refined the treatment method and applied it not only to back injury and back pain but to neck injury and neck pain. Most specifically, I have identified seven powerful exercises for the back and seven more for the neck. The method, which also includes postural correction, has become known as the McKenzie Method. Medical researchers have verified the effectiveness of the method for both diagnosis and treatment. Many research articles, published in professional journals, support the method's techniques.

The main features of the human spine are the vertebrae—small bony structures that are separated and cushioned by the discs. Distortion of the discs—changes in their shape—often causes pain in the back and neck. The exercises I have developed allow the discs to return to their normal shape. The result is that pain disappears.

The exciting thing is that sometimes the pain disappears almost instantly. In some ways, the exercises appeal to the energetic and dedicated: these exercises are for people who want to stop depending 100 percent on others—health professionals—to take care of them. But at the same time, the exercises may also appeal to the lazy.

The exercises are easy to do. Certain important exercises require the reader to hold a position for about two seconds and repeat the exercise five to ten times. Each exercise session will last no longer than 60 seconds from start to finish. In the early stages of the program, exercise sessions should be repeated seven or eight times a day. To remain pain-free for life, readers will need to adopt good posture (even that becomes a comfortable thing to do over time) and perform the exercises twice daily—just two minutes out of their day.

THE PROBLEM

Back pain and neck pain are serious business and big business. They are serious business because they are vexing: many back pain "sufferers" really are suffering a great deal. Their pain is severe, sometimes disabling, often distracting. Sometimes it shoots down their legs (this is called *sciatica*). Neck pain can in at least one sense be even worse than back pain: being so close to the head, it's a very personal pain. Like a headache, it's hard—if not impossible—to ignore. It too can be disabling.

If you have back pain or neck pain, you may have had to stop playing sports. If your back pain is bad enough, you may not even be able to walk. Either back or neck pain may have kept you home from work.

It may surprise you to know that back pain and neck pain are related. Most neck sufferers also have or will have back pain, and a large percentage of back sufferers also have or will have neck pain. Due to problems such as poor posture, a man or woman with back pain is more likely to develop neck pain than is a person without back trouble.

Despite the magnitude of the problem, most people do not get adequate and cost-effective treatment for their back or neck pain. They continue to suffer month after month, year after year.

Chronic lower back pain is probably the most extensive and costly medical problem in the world. It seems that everyone has back pain. The consensus, based on many scientific studies, is that during their lifetimes more than 80 percent of the people in Western nations suffer at least one episode of back pain severe enough to require bed rest; many others experience back pain that is troubling if not severe. Studies indicate that neck pain presents a severe problem at least once in the lives of 40 percent of the population of these countries.

So back and neck pain are *serious* business. But how are they *big* business? In just the U.S., back pain costs from $50 billion to $70 billion a year in everything from medical expenses to days lost from work.

Most people who suffer back and neck pain struggle along on their own. But some visit an orthopedist for an appointment where the chief beneficiary is the doctor, who may bill $275 for an initial examination. In return for this, the physician often gives the patient nothing more than two prescription slips, one for drugs (which in some cases are ineffective or have unpleasant side effects, or both) and another providing a vague but expensive referral to physical therapy. If drugs and physical therapy don't do the trick, some physicians recommend surgery.

Sometimes surgery is successful; sometimes it is not. All back and neck surgery is costly and requires a recovery period of several weeks, during which time most patients cannot go to work. Most surgery helps more than it hurts, but some operations reduce only some of a patient's pain, and other surgeries are completely unsuccessful: range of motion is reduced and pain is not.

Physical therapists and chiropractors may bill $100 per appointment for several appointments a week over many consecutive months. The bill can easily mount well into the thousands of dollars. These well-meaning professionals may do little more than briefly reduce pain through what they call *modalities*, but which are nothing more sophisticated or effective than ice, heat, and ultrasound. And who has so much leisure time that he or she can easily find three hours a week for treatment, plus the time it takes to get to and from the therapist?

If you are a typical person suffering back pain, you have recurring pain. The attacks are not getting less frequent; they may even be occurring more often. They may be more disabling than they once were.

Or your problem may not be recurring, rather, it may be bothering you nearly every day, month after month, in which case it is *chronic*. Very likely, it has not responded well to physical therapy, chiropractic care, or medication— whether over-the-counter (OTC) or prescription.

Or you may have had surgery for your back or neck. Even though you went to a qualified surgeon, the surgery may well have failed to correct your problem.

Every year for 35 years I saw a thousand patients. These patients taught me that the only people who really needed my services were those with recurrent or chronic back problems. The rest would get better on their own and stay better for long periods. My thousands of patients also taught me that most of them, and therefore most back and neck patients in general, could learn to manage their own problems once they were taught the right exercises, the exercises I describe in this book.

I even found that despite my best efforts, which conformed to the care given by the best physical therapists in my country and others, I was *getting in the way* of finding out which patients could successfully treat themselves. It became clear that if I used the usual "modalities"—heat, ultrasound, spinal manipulation, or spinal adjustment—and the patient got better, I had at least temporarily eliminated the opportunity to see if exercise was enough.

So it became evident that not only were the exercises a great help to the great majority of patients, but that they should be used very early in the treatment of patients. In this way, we could identify the many who could "cure themselves" through exercise at home and the few who did require "hands-on" treatment by a physical therapist or other health practitioner.

Once they were taught self-management, most patients with recurring or chronic problems would willingly shoulder (no pun intended) the responsibility for their own care. Many had lost all hope that they would ever be free of back or neck pain. Many had come to assume that the only relief, even if it was only temporary, would come at the expensive hands of a health care expert. But now they were in charge of their own problem.

They had become used to driving to the office of the physical therapist or chiropractor or physician, waiting to be called into the treatment room, partially undressing, having the health professional "work on them," and driving back to their jobs or homes. These visits, travel included, would take hours every week, and sometimes hundreds of hours a year, that could be put to other use. The patients had become used to seeing large amounts of money transferred to the health professional's office or health maintenance organization—their money, or an insurance company's money, or some combination. They had believed they were in a dark, endless tunnel lined with time and money.

Now the patients learned the exercises. They found they were effective. They found they took very little time, a tiny fraction of the time it would take for an appointment. They found they were easy to do. And so they found a light at the end of the tunnel!

Lower back pain affects nearly all of us at some stage of our active adult life. It is therefore one of the most common health problems afflicting mankind. It can follow an event or can just accompany aging (and I'm not talking about old age here: many people first encounter recurring or chronic back pain in their thirties, and a sizable number encounter it much earlier). It can be called by many names. Among these are fibrositis, fibromyalgia, slipped disc, degenerative disc disease, arthritis of the lower back, rheumatism, lumbago. When the pain extends into the leg, it is called sciatica.

To most people with lower back pain, the cause of their pain is a mystery. Often it starts without warning and for no obvious reason. It interferes with the most simple activities of living, activities that, until the back pain began, the person took for granted. Activities as simple as walking, sitting, and standing. Less simple activities, such as participating in sports or driving a car or participating in family events, become less pleasant or even unpleasant; often they are avoided. Lower back pain also interferes with the critical "non-activity" of getting a good night's sleep.

Then, just as unexpectedly, the pain subsides or disappears entirely. When in acute (recent, sharp) pain, we are usually unable to think in a calm, deliberate manner about our trouble. Our mind is focused on getting relief. On the other hand, as soon as we have recovered from an acute episode, most of us quickly forget our lower back problems. (Certainly there are other things to think about, other responsibilities to undertake!)

Therefore, once we have developed recurring back pain, we can do nothing but seek assistance, time and again, to become pain-free. Due to a lack of knowledge and understanding, we've been unable to deal with symptoms when they are present, and until now we have had no way of preventing future symptoms.

THE SOLUTION

You can stop your own back pain and neck pain.

You may have thought that your options were limited to these six:

1. going to a doctor
2. going to a physical therapist
3. going to a chiropractor
4. using prescription or over-the-counter drugs
5. some combination of the above, or
6. doing nothing and hoping the pain will just go away.

In fact, there is a powerful seventh alternative: *you can take care of yourself.* Through simple exercises I explain in this book, you can eliminate—or at least dramatically reduce—your back or neck pain in a matter of minutes.

Mr. Smith gave us the discovery of the power of extension. We have built upon it, and now the McKenzie Method is much more than that. In particular, it includes a method of assessment of patients that can be used by health professionals. But even after decades of development, the heart of the McKenzie Method is still extension: bending or pushing the back or neck into a straight position or past it. Extension is the opposite of *flexion*, the position that most people assume when sitting or standing at work or leisure. Poor posture, in which people are too often in flexion, is the most common cause of back and neck injury.

We have developed wonderfully easy and effective sets of seven exercises for the back and seven for the neck that challenge such mottos as "You get what you pay for" and "No pain, no gain." The exercises are quick and easy to perform. Most people benefit dramatically from performing only one or two to the seven exercises. The full array of exercises provides a range of weapons for attacking pain and stiffness in the back and neck, as well as providing a person with the tools to reduce the risk of future episodes.

One need not do all seven exercises for either the neck or the back. Most people benefit dramatically from doing only a few. In a session lasting only a few minutes, many will experience great relief.

While the McKenzie Method is best known for extension, several of its exercises involve flexion. As a result, the exercises provide a full range of weapons for attacking pain and stiffness in the back and neck.

The other major contribution of the method is this advice to back and neck sufferers: *treat yourself.* The norm in Western nations is that if you have a medical problem, you see a doctor or other health professional. Yet we have found that the great majority of back and neck sufferers can treat themselves successfully without ever walking into a health professional's office. They can treat themselves successfully through the McKenzie exercises.

Fortunately, there has been movement toward the method. In particular, U.S. federal guidelines from the Agency for Health Care Policy and Research approve of movement, minimal bedrest, patient education, and self-responsibility. (Bios, S. et al., "Acute low back problems in adults: clinical practice guidelines, quick reference guide no. 14," 1994, U.S. Department of Health and Human Services, Agency for Health Care Policy and Research; Rockville, MD.)

The causes of most kinds of common lower back problems are quite clear. First, I will explain why lower back pain may occur. Then I will suggest how you can avoid it. Or, if you are having lower back pain right now, I will suggest how you may recover from it and what steps you can take if it reappears.

The main point of this book is that the management of your back is *your responsibility.* Of course, you can call on people with particular skills—doctors, physical therapists, or chiropractors—for treatment. But in the end, *only you can really help yourself.* That is, only you can help yourself become pain-free not only *during* clinical appointments but *without* appointments. Self-treatment of lower back pain is now widely recommended; it will be more effective in the long-term management of your lower back problems than any other form of treatment.

Dozens of books set out to tell you how to care for your own back, so you may wonder why yet another one is now offered. The reason is that this is the first book ever offered in U.S. bookstores that shows you how to *put your back in* if you are unfortunate enough to have *put it out.* In addition, this book shows you what steps you must take to avoid recurrence.

If you have developed lower back pain or neck pain for the first time, consult a health care professional such as your family doctor, a physical therapist who frequently treats back or neck pain, or a chiropractor. Also seek the advice of such a health care professional if there are complications to your lower back pain; for example, if you have constant pain that travels down your leg all the way to your foot, if you have numbness, if you have muscle weakness, or if, in addition to having back pain, you feel unwell. All these circumstances indicate the need to consult a health professional. If you are not sure whether you should consult such a professional, err on the side of protecting yourself and consult one.

The McKenzie Institute International has provided education and training in the McKenzie Method to more than 20,000 physical therapists, chiropractors, and physicians around the world. In the event that the exercises and other advice in this book fail to give you sufficient relief from your back or neck problem, consult a health practitioner trained in the McKenzie Method. Being intimately familiar with the McKenzie exercises, these professionals are uniquely qualified to determine whether exercises should be enough to provide you with relief or whether more traditional, "hands-on" means are appropriate. (Indeed, in a relatively small minority of cases, the exercises are not enough.) Very often, a one-on-one session with an expert trained in the McKenzie Method will clarify the nature of your problem and the steps you must take to resolve it.

To find a McKenzie-trained health professional in your area, please see Appendix A: How to Find a McKenzie-Trained Health Care Practitioner, near the end of this book.

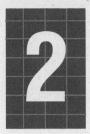

2 How Your Back and Neck Work and Why They Hurt

THE CULPRIT: BAD POSTURE

By far the most common cause of back pain and neck pain is poor posture. Therefore, back pain often follows the following actions:

- Sitting for a long time

- Bending for a long period or over and over—usually at work

- Lifting heavy objects

- Standing

- Lying down in a position of strain

Similarly, neck pain often follows poor posture in activities such as these:

- Sitting for a long period

- Working in a strained position (such as the office worker who often holds a phone in place between the head and shoulder, or the tractor operator who often rotates his head to look behind him)

- Lying down or sleeping with the head in an awkward position.

This book will help you maintain good posture and will allow you to eliminate the pain and stiffness that come from bad posture.

Lordosis

Before you begin the exercises, you must understand what bad posture is. And to do that, you must understand the meaning of the word *lordosis*. To some, this term may sound like a disease or an abnormal condition. In fact, it is a natural feature of the lumbar spine in all people.

A lordosis is an inward curve of the spine. The inward curve in the lower back is called the *lumbar lordosis* (Fig. 2.5). This lordosis is found in the small of the back, just above the waistline. Some people refer to it as the "hollow" in the lower back. The smaller inward curve in the neck is called the *cervical lordosis*.

When a person stands upright, the lordosis naturally occurs. Still, the degree of lordosis varies from person to person and from activity to activity.

Maintenance of the lumbar lordosis isn't just valuable in the effort to make the back healthy and pain-free: it is *critical*. Nevertheless, even though the lordosis is natural and despite its importance, it is not always present in all people. In fact, almost everyone loses the lordosis during certain activities, such as bending over and touching one's toes.

The lordosis is lost whenever the lower back is "rounded," as usually occurs when people sit or when they bend forward. And if the lordosis is lost often or for long periods or both, lower back problems frequently result.

ANATOMY

To understand *why* back problems can result from loss of the lordosis, let's quickly focus on human anatomy.

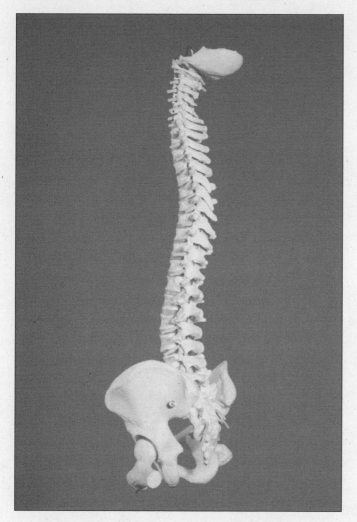

Figure 2.1 *The human spine viewed from the side.*

The spine or "backbone" (Fig. 2.1) is made up of vertebrae. Each vertebra looks something like a spool of thread (Fig. 2.2). It is circular and has a hole that runs from top to bottom. There are 33 vertebrae (Fig. 2.1): seven in the neck (the *cervical vertebrae*), 12 in the upper back (the *thoracic vertebrae*), five in the lower back (the *lumbar vertebrae*), five fused together in the sacrum (the *sacral vertebrae*), and four rudimentary vertebrae fused together in the coccyx (the *coccygeal vertebrae*; these are the lowest part of the spine and are the vestige of a tail).

With the vertebrae lined up one atop the other, the holes form the spinal canal (Fig. 2.3). Through this canal runs the bundle of nerves that extends from the head to the pelvis—the spinal cord.

Between each pair of vertebrae are two small openings through which the left and right spinal nerves leave the spinal canal (Fig. 2.4). Among other things, these nerves give power to the muscles and give sensation to the skin. It is through the spinal nerves that you can move and can feel temperature,

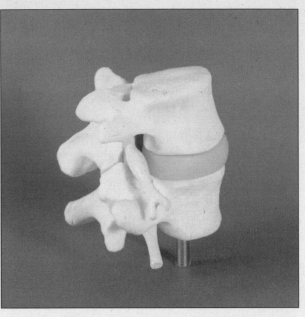

Figure 2.2 *The vertebrae are similar to a stack of cotton spools.*

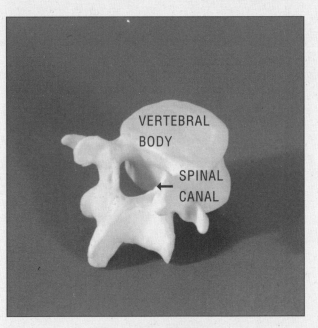

VERTEBRAL BODY

SPINAL CANAL

Figure 2.3 *A vertebra*

pressure, and pain. These sensations are not just normal parts of life; they also provide a natural alarm system: they warn you that a bodily structure is about to sustain some damage or has already been damaged.

In the lower part of the spine, some of the left and right spinal nerves combine to form the left and right sciatic nerves, which serve the legs. When these nerves are compressed or irritated, they can cause pain in the leg. The pain often extends below the knee. Pain extending from the lower back to below the knee is called *sciatica*.

Between the spool-like vertebrae are special structures made out of cartilage, a dense connective tissue capable of withstanding considerable pressure. In the human body, there are three types of cartilage: *hyaline cartilage, elastic cartilage,* and *fibrocartilage.* The type found in the spine is fibrocartilage.

Intervertebral discs are special cartilage structures between the vertebrae. Just as the vertebrae are similar to spools, the discs are similar to rubber washers, round and made of a flexible material; unlike

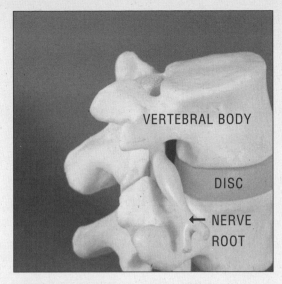

VERTEBRAL BODY

DISC

← NERVE ROOT

Figure 2.4   Two vertebrae

many washers, however, they don't have a hole in the middle.

The semi-fluid center of the disc is called the *nucleus pulposus*, "nucleus" for short. Surrounding the nucleus is a cartilage ring, called the *annulus* or annular ligament.

The discs are the shock absorbers of the spine. They are flexible enough that they can alter their shape, allowing one vertebra to move on another and allowing movement of the back as a whole.

The vertebrae and discs of the lower back form the lumbar spine and are linked by a series of joints. Each joint is held together by soft tissues that surround it. These tissues are reinforced by *ligaments*, tough bands of fibrous connective tissue. The ligaments that reinforce the capsule that surrounds a spinal joint are like guy wires that support an outdoor television antenna by pulling on it and attaching it to the roof. The spinal ligaments strengthen the joint and limit its movement to certain directions.

Then there are the muscles, which lie over one or more joints of the lower back. The muscles extend upward to the trunk and downward to the pelvis. At each end, each muscle becomes a tendon, which attaches the muscle to one or more bones. When a muscle contracts, it causes movement in one or more joints.

BETTER TO BE A QUADRUPED THAN A HUMAN?

Humans descended from four-legged animals but in most ways are more advanced. Few lions or monkeys are good chess players. But, when contrasted to humans, lions and monkeys also have spines that are far less likely to become painful. In animals that walk on all fours, the weight of the body is distributed evenly over the four legs. Most of the time the spine is held in a more or less horizontal position. The forces that compress the human spine simply do not exist.

In human beings, however, the spine is held in a more-or-less vertical position—at least during waking and working hours. When you are upright, the lumbar spine bears the weight of the entire body above it. This weight compresses the spine. The lumbar spine also transmits this weight to the pelvis when you sit, and to the feet when you stand, walk, or run.

The lumbar spine, providing a flexible connection between the upper and lower halves of the body, protects the spinal cord. It also has a greater function in weight-bearing in humans than it does in quadrupeds. In the evolution of the horizontal-spine posture of animals to the vertical-spine posture of man, the discs between the vertebrae have adapted to support heavier weights. In addition, the spinal column has developed a series of curves that ingeniously allow for better shock absorption and flexibility.

LOSS OF LORDOSIS

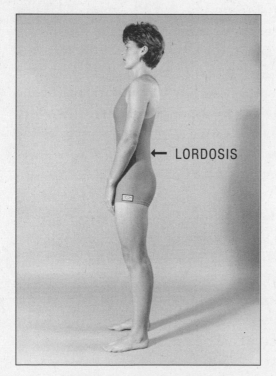

← LORDOSIS

Figure 2.5 Lumbar lordosis

Remember the lordosis? That's the natural inward curve, or hollow, in the small of the back (Fig. 2.5). When you stand upright, the lordosis is naturally present. You lose the lordosis when you sit or bend forward. And if you lose the lordosis often or for long periods or both, you can suffer problems of the lower back. In particular, you can suffer problems in the ligaments that act as guy wires supporting and reinforcing the capsule of tissues that surround and hold together the spinal joints. When these ligaments become fatigued or overstretched, pain often results.

MECHANICAL PAIN

Once you have become familiar with this section and the one titled "Mechanical Lower Back Pain," at the beginning of the next chapter, you will be more than halfway toward solving your back and neck pain problems. Research has shown that the better a person understands the problems that cause back or neck pain, the more effectively he or she can treat himself or herself. In particular, the person learns why the exercises in this book are effective and how to do these exercises. Further, he or she is more highly motivated to maintain the exercise program.

Mechanical pain occurs when the joint between two bones anywhere in the body has been placed in a position that overstretches the surrounding ligaments and other soft tissues.

To help understand how easily some mechanical pains can be produced, try this experiment:

1. Slowly bend a finger backward (Fig. 2.6). Bend it until you feel a *strain*. If you leave the finger in the strained position, at first you will feel only minor discomfort. But as time passes, substantial *pain* will eventually develop. Sometimes this will take as long as an hour.

2. Repeat the experiment, but with a change. This time, bend the finger past the point of *strain* until you feel *pain*. The sensation of pain is immediate. In this case, you have overstretched, and your pain is acting as an alarm system. It is telling you that to continue movement in the current direction will cause damage.

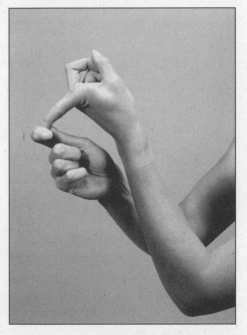

Figure 2.6
Bend the finger until you feel the strain.

The ligaments and surrounding soft tissues that hold the joint together would be torn, resulting in an ache that would continue even when the finger was at rest. This pain would increase with movement and decline at rest, but it would not cease until some healing had occurred. Healing would take several days but would be prolonged if, day after day, you continued to apply the same strains to the finger.

Just as one can experience pain or damage in the finger, one can suffer pain or damage in the back or neck. Holding the neck or back in the wrong position can cause a lot of pain, and holding the back or neck in a position past the point of strain will cause injury.

Most people can sit with poor posture for some period of time without suffering damage or pain. But over time—during a single afternoon or after years of poor posture—the result in most people will eventually be pain and stiffness in the back or neck or both.

We are already doing our best to cause ourselves back and neck trouble. But we are not without help. Our accomplices in the effort to cause ourselves pain through poor posture are the manufacturers of furniture in homes and seats in motor vehicles. Examples of stationary furniture can be found in the home and in the office: kitchen chairs, dining room chairs, lounge chairs, couches, and sofas.

Furniture that moves generally is attached to a car or van or truck. The most common culprit is the car seat. Whether it sits still or moves along at freeway speeds, your seating furniture is probably doing its best to hurt your back and neck.

Bad chairs and bad car seats seem to have been designed by people who own too many rulers: there are too many straight lines. But people's backs and necks contain curves. In particular, there is the lumbar lordosis, which must be maintained if back pain is to be prevented. A seat back that is straight does nothing to maintain the lordosis, and it encourages you to sit in the very slouch that, unfortunately, you are quite capable of producing by yourself.

In addition to having seat backs that are straight, most bad chairs and seats have one other thing in common: they slant backward. Such chairs don't just make it nearly impossible to maintain good posture; these chairs almost *mandate* that the sitter become a sloucher.

But there are alternatives.

First, you can look for good chairs and good car seats. In every case, whether in an office or an automobile, good seats will include an outward curve near the bottom of the seat back. If it is in the right position or if it is adjustable to the right position, this curve will fit into the lordosis, supporting it. Second, if you are stuck with a chair or car seat that looks better than it feels, you can still do something about it. In particular, you can add something to provide the support your lower back needs. For the back, the best device to add is a firm foam rubber lumbar roll.

Certain lumbar rolls are especially effective in helping to avert and treat pain and stiffness in the back. The best design is found not only in the roll's shape but in the precise density and quality of the foam rubber it contains. The best type of lumbar roll comes with an adjustable strap that fits around the back of most any chair or car seat. Until you can get yourself a lumbar roll, try rolling up a bath towel or beach towel or even using a paper towel roll.

Although the lumbar roll of course fits into the lumbar spine, it helps the cervical spine too. It is the opposite of a pain in the neck: it helps to *avoid* a pain in the neck. In supporting the lower back, the lumbar support helps straighten the spine. This in turn naturally causes the posture of the neck to improve, so that the neck is more in a straight line with the rest of the spine. As the neck becomes more in line with the spine, the head retracts. The neck itself is therefore in a more healthful position, and it is not straining by supporting a head that is protruding forward.

There are also well-designed rolls for the neck, called cervical rolls. They are smaller than the lumbar roll but also made of a special foam rubber. The cervical roll is designed to provide proper support of the neck when you lie down to rest or sleep.

Remember, by correcting your lower back posture you also begin the correction of your neck posture. Then, when you simply tuck in your chin while keeping your head and eyes level, your head and neck will be in the proper position, and you will be on your way to stopping your pain.

The better the posture of your back, neck, and head, the faster your pain will go away.

ANATOMY AND EXERCISE

In Chapter 5, you will learn the seven simple exercises that will help you rapidly stop your back symptoms. In Chapter 12, you will learn the seven simple exercises that will help you quickly eliminate your neck pain. But it may help you to understand the anatomy behind the exercises.

Not all exercises in this book work in the same way, but many are designed to change the shape of the distorted disc. The distortion is often *posterior*, meaning there is a bulge toward the back of the nucleus of the disc and in the back of the *annulus*, the outer wall that surrounds the nucleus. The bulge causes pain either because the annulus itself contains nerves or because the bulging disc pushes on the spinal nerves. Many of the exercises put the sufferer in "extension," the opposite of "flexion," the forward-bending posture that caused the distortion. Extension causes a tilt in certain adjacent vertebrae, reducing the space between the back parts. This pushes the disc nucleus *anteriorly*, or forward. In this situation, you can move the nucleus easily, like a person with wet hands squeezing a bar of soap. The forward movement of the disc reduces or eliminates the posterior bulge. The result? Your pain is gone.

Back Problems

MECHANICAL LOWER BACK PAIN

If an engineer were to determine which part of the back was subjected to the greatest mechanical stress, he or she would name the part of the spine just above the pelvis—the lumbar spine. The lower the part of the spine, the more weight it supports. Below the lumbar spine are the *coccyx* and *sacrum*, whose vertebrae don't move and therefore cannot be placed in the wrong position. But the vertebrae of the *lumbar* spine do move and can move into the wrong position; in particular, they can lose their lordosis (their inward curve). In naming the lumbar spine as the focus of the greatest mechanical stress, the engineer would be right, because the lumbar spine is the lowest part of the spine that can move and because statistics show that back problems arise more often in the lower back than in any other part of the spine.

People once believed that pain in the back and neck was caused by drafts, chills, or the weather. But we now know that it is generally caused by mechanical strains of the type described in the previous chapter.

Many people think back and neck pain is caused by muscle strain. Occasionally this is the case. Muscles can indeed be overstretched or injured. But this requires a considerable amount of force and does not happen often. Moreover, muscles usually heal very rapidly and seldom cause pain lasting for more than a week or two.

In fact, most pain in the back and neck is caused by prolonged over-stretching of ligaments and other surrounding soft tissues. Just as pain arises in the overstretched finger, pain can arise in the back and neck when ligaments are overstretched.

The most common cause of pain from overstretching is *poor posture*. Whenever you remain in a relaxed position, whether standing, sitting, or lying down, prolonged overstretching can easily occur.

Most people slouch. That's the bad news, but it's also the good news. If the problem was caused only by another person or by a disease, there might be little you could do to prevent it. But since you are the cause, you have control over the problem.

More good news: The strain brought on by prolonged overstretching can easily be avoided. And once you have read this book, you not only will know that you must take responsibility for your posture, but you also will know how to maintain good posture. Further, you will know how to exercise to eliminate pain.

Another source of significant lower back and neck pain is severe over-stretching of supporting ligaments. Severe overstretching may occur when an outside force places an excessive strain on the back or neck. This type of strain can occur due to a collision in a contact sport, from a fall while playing tennis, or while lifting excessive weight. Other examples of damaging forces are auto accidents and industrial accidents. None of these types of injury can easily be avoided, as they typically occur unexpectedly, without warning signs.

When soft tissues surrounding a joint are overstretched, it is usually the ligaments that first cause pain. Overstretching of the spinal joints causes special problems, because the ligaments that surround these joints also act as retaining walls for the spinal discs. As explained, these discs are the shock absorbers of the spine. Overstretching the spinal ligaments can affect the discs. This may affect the intensity of the pain you feel, the distribution of the pain, and the behavior of the pain. The pain may become better or worse with certain movements or positions.

Sometimes the ligament is injured to such an extent that the disc loses its ability to absorb shock and its outer wall (annulus) is weakened. Once the outer wall is weakened, the soft inside of the disc (the nucleus) bulges outward, often pressing on the spinal nerves and causing pain. Sometimes mere distortion of the outer wall causes pain without impinging on the spinal nerve, because the annulus itself contains nerves.

In extreme cases, the nucleus will burst through this outer wall, which may cause severe pain. If the disc bulges far enough backward, it will press painfully on the sciatic nerve. This can cause pain or other problems (numbness, a sensation of "pins and needles," weakness) to be felt far from the source of trouble—as far away as the lower leg or foot.

If the disc nucleus bulges excessively, the disc may become severely distorted. This will cause the vertebrae to tilt forward or to one side and will prevent the vertebrae from lining up properly during movement. In this case, some movements will be blocked partially or completely, and any movement may cause acute pain.

When acute back pain develops, people often stand with the trunk off-center or bent forward. If you experience a sudden onset of pain and, following this, are unable to straighten up or move the back properly, you are likely to have some bulging in the disc nucleus. As bad as this may sound, *this need not be cause for alarm*. The exercises in this book are carefully designed to reduce any disturbance of this nature.

If you have caused damage to soft tissues, you will feel some pain until your healing is complete and your function is fully restored. During the healing process it is important that you avoid movements that pull the healing surfaces apart. For example, if you have overstretched the ligaments of the lower back by bending forward, it is likely that any repetition of this movement will continue to open and separate the healing tissues, and this will delay healing. If, on the other hand, you avoid bending forward and instead retain the hollow (the lumbar lordosis) in the lower back, the damaged surfaces will remain together and healing will not be interrupted. In the same way, if your pain is in the neck, it is important that you avoid bending your neck forward and instead retain the smaller hollow (the cervical lordosis) in your neck.

To illustrate, let's again use the finger, but in a different way. Instead of focusing on overstretching the finger, let's imagine that you have cut your finger across the back of the knuckle. If you were to bend the injured finger joint every day, you would open up the wound and delay healing. But if you were to keep the finger straight for about a week, you would allow the healing surfaces to stay together, and complete healing would result. Once healing was complete, you could bend the finger without risking further damage. Similarly, if you maintain the correct posture and allow your back or neck to heal, you will be able to resume normal bending of each without damage or pain.

But there's more. When tissues heal, they form scar tissue, which is less elastic than normal tissue and tends to shorten over time. If shortening has occurred, movement may stretch the scars and cause pain. Unless appropriate exercises are performed to restore normal flexibility, the healed tissues may become a continuous source of pain or stiffness, or both, in the back or neck. Such problems may persist for years. Even though the original damage has repaired, the scar itself may restrict movement and cause pain when overstretched.

Where Is the Pain Felt?

The location of pain caused by lower back problems varies from one person to another. In a first attack of back pain, the pain is usually felt at or around the beltline. It may be felt in the center of the back (Fig. 3.1) or just to one side (Fig. 3.2). Usually, the pain declines within a few days.

In later attacks, pain may extend as far as the buttock (Fig. 3.3). In still later episodes, the pain may go all the way to the back or outside of the thigh and on down to the knee (Fig. 3.4). It may even extend to the ankle or foot (Fig. 3.5). Less frequently, pain may be felt in the front of the thigh, down to the knee (Fig. 3.6).

The pain may vary with your movements or with the positions in which you place your body. Its intensity may change. Or its location may vary. For example, one movement may result in buttock pain, while another may eliminate the pain in the buttock, only for the pain to relocate to the lower back.

If your problem is severe, you may have not only pain but other symptoms. In particular, you may experience significant numbness in the lower leg or find that you have muscular weakness in the same place.

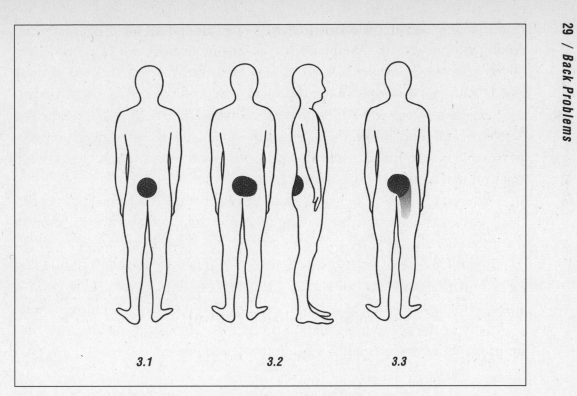

Figures 3.1–3.3 *Sites of pain caused by lower back problems*

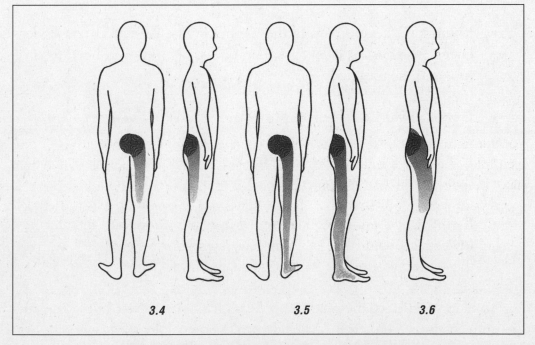

Figures 3.4–3.6 *Sites of pain caused by lower back problems*

WHO CAN PERFORM SELF-TREATMENT?

Most people with back pain will benefit from the advice in this book. And most people with this pain can immediately start our exercise program—provided that the precautions below are followed. The McKenzie Method program is generally effective, but it is not for every person. It is safe for all, provided that this book's precautions are carried out and that its questions are answered accurately.

Once you start the exercises, carefully observe whether your pain is getting better, getting worse, or staying the same, and whether the location of the pain is changing.

In particular, if your pain was getting worse before you started the exercises and does not improve after the first two days, *seek advice from a health professional* such as a physician, physical therapist, or chiropractor.

If any of the following situations occurs, do *not* begin our exercise program without first consulting a health professional:

- If you have developed lower back pain for the first time and it is no better 10 days after onset

- If you have severe pain in the leg below the knee and you experience sensations of weakness, numbness, or "pins and needles" in a foot and the toes

- If your lower back problems followed a recent severe accident

- If, following a recent severe episode of back pain, you have developed bladder problems

- If you are generally feeling unwell in conjunction with the attack of lower back pain (that is, if you have symptoms other than back pain that began around the same time as the back pain)

To help you determine whether you can treat your lower back pain successfully without help from a health professional, please answer the following questions:

- Are there periods in the day—even as short as ten minutes—when you have no pain?

- Is the pain confined to areas above the knee?

- Are you generally worse when sitting for prolonged periods or when standing up from the sitting position?

- Are you generally worse during or right after prolonged bending or stooping, as when making a bed, vacuuming, ironing, gardening, or laying concrete?

- Are you generally worse when getting up in the morning, but improve after about half an hour?

- Are you generally worse when inactive and better when on the move?

- Are you generally better when walking?

- Are you generally better when lying facedown? When testing this, you may feel worse for the first few minutes but then feel better; in this case, the answer to this question is yes.

- Have you had several episodes of lower back pain over the past months or years?

If you have answered yes to all the questions, you are an ideal candidate for the self-treatment program outlined in this book. But we're not hard graders here: there are nine questions above, but if you have answered yes to only four or more of them, you have a good chance of benefitting from the program and you should begin it.

Even if you have answered yes to three or fewer of the nine questions, it's possible you will benefit from the program. But to determine whether this is the case, consult a health professional trained in or, ideally, credentialed in, the McKenzie Method. This provider can help you determine whether you can start the program or if, instead of our program (or in addition to it), you require a form of specialized treatment that only a health professional can provide. To obtain the names of credentialed members and associates of the McKenzie Institute, please see Appendix A: How to Find a McKenzie-Trained Health Care Practitioner, which appears at the back of this book.

If you have answered yes to zero to three of the above questions, it may be that at least for the moment the distortion in the affected joint is too great to be reduced effectively by self-treatment alone. In that case, ideally you will see a practitioner trained in the McKenzie method.

Common Causes of Lower Back Pain

POSTURAL CAUSES

The most common cause of lower back pain is postural stress. For this reason, lower back pain frequently is brought on by sitting for a long time in a poor position (Fig. 4.1), by prolonged bending in a bad working position (Fig. 4.2), by heavy lifting (Fig. 4.3), or by standing (Fig. 4.4) or lying down for a long time in a poor position. When you look carefully at the accompanying photographs, you will see that the lower back is rounded and that the all-important lordosis—the inward curve or hollow in the lumbar spine—has disappeared.

Unfortunately, many people lose the lordosis much of the time each day and seldom if ever increase it to its very maximum. If you reduce the lordosis for long periods at a time, year in and year out, and you never properly restore it, you will eventually lose your ability to form the hollow. The clinical experience of countless health professionals has demonstrated that a flattened lower back often is associated with chronic lower back problems.

When they walk or run, most people naturally have a lordosis in the lower back. As a result, these activities frequently help to relieve lower back pain. Also, when we are standing, the lordosis naturally is present. But in some individuals, when the standing posture is maintained for a long time, the lordosis becomes excessive and pain will result.

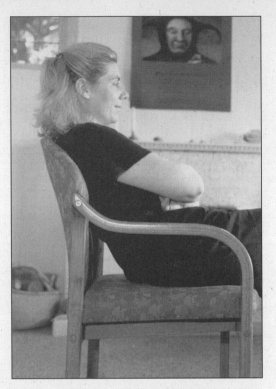

Figure 4.1   *Poor sitting position*

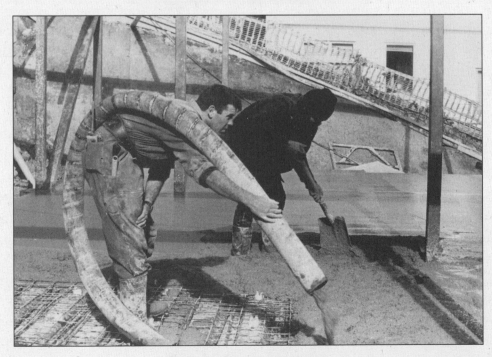

Figure 4.2   *Bad working position*

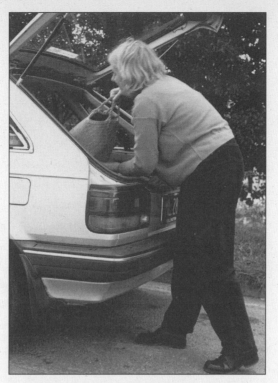

Figure 4.3 *Poor lifting technique*

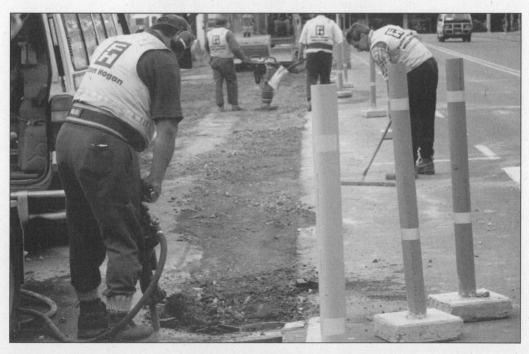

Figure 4.4 *Standing in poor position*

But of all the many postural stresses that can result in pain, by far the worst is poor sitting posture. A poor sitting posture may by itself produce lower back pain. Once lower back problems have developed, a poor sitting posture will in all likelihood perpetuate or worsen these problems.

Other frequent causes of back pain include poor standing postures and poor lying postures. You may know this already, because you may already have found that your back pain appears only if you stand for long periods or only after you get into bed. Pain that behaves in this way frequently is caused by poor posture alone. If this is your situation, you're in luck, because this type of pain can easily be eliminated.

If you have poor posture in sitting, standing, or lying down, you will not have pain if you avoid prolonged overstretching. If pain does develop, it's an almost certain indication that you have poor posture and that you must immediately take steps to correct it. Once you have determined what your postural problem is and how to correct it, you should not have to seek assistance from a health professional every time postural pain arises; rather, you should be able to treat yourself rapidly, easily, and effectively.

Consequences of Postural Neglect

Some people who habitually adopt poor posture remain unaware that their posture is causing their back pain. These people experience back pain throughout their lifetime simply because they do not have the information needed to correct the postural faults.

When pains stemming from bad posture are first felt, they are easily eliminated if one merely corrects his or her posture. But if time passes and posture is not corrected, the habitual poor posture causes changes in structure and shape of the joints. As a result, excessive wear occurs in the joints and the joints age prematurely. As a further consequence, the effects of poor posture can be just as severe and just as harmful as the effects of an injury.

Those of us who permit poor posture to persist throughout our lifetimes become bent and stooped as the aging process develops. If we are in this situation, and we are called upon to straighten and stand erect, we cannot do so, much as we might like to. For many of us in this situation, if we are asked to turn the head, we cannot do this either. Our mobility is now so impaired that we appear to others to be old, because we exhibit the postures and mobility problems of the elderly.

Stooped posture and restrictions in mobility are the *visible* effects of poor posture that has become habitual. But there are also secondary consequences to the *organs* that may be even more severe, invisible as they are to others. As the back becomes bent, the lungs may become constricted, and as a result our breathing may be affected. The stomach and other internal organs may be deprived of their correct support and may function less effectively than otherwise would be the case.

The typical person believes that the bent, stooped posture seen in so many of our older friends and relatives is an inevitable consequence of aging. This is not the case. And I believe the time to commence preventive action is *now*. If only *once a day* we stand fully erect and bend fully backward, we need never lose the ability to perform those actions and therefore we need never become bent, stooped, and impaired in how we look and in how our bodies function internally.

1. SITTING FOR LONG PERIODS

Poor posture in sitting is by far the most common cause of pain and stiffness in the back and, for that matter, in the neck. Most everyone spends a great deal of time sitting: even if you do not spend most of your day behind a desk, you probably spend much of your evening in an easy chair or on a couch. *Most* people who sit for long periods will eventually develop poor posture in sitting. This is because when you sit in a particular position for even a few minutes, the muscles that support your lower back and your neck become tired. When they become tired, you relax, placing yourself in a position of poor posture.

Your body sags. You slouch in a chair, adopting a position that is still sitting, but is somewhere between sitting straight up and lying down. As a result, you typically lose the lordosis in the back and the lordosis in the neck.

If you stay in a slouched sitting posture long enough, your ligaments will become overstretched and pain and stiffness will result. Worse, once the slouched sitting posture has become a habit and is maintained most of the time, it may also cause distortion of the nucleus of the discs in the vertebral joints. (A distorted disc is one that has lost its normal shape; typically, it bulges in one direction or another.) Once this occurs, pain will come not only from certain positions but from certain movements.

Poor sitting posture may itself produce lower back pain. And, regardless of the original cause, once lower back pain or stiffness has developed, poor sitting posture will perpetuate or worsen the problem.

It follows that people with office jobs that involve a lot of sitting easily develop lower back problems, because many sit with a rounded back—a back not maintaining the lordosis—for hours on end. If you are an office worker, you may go through the following stages of gradually increasing back problems, unless you take steps to rectify the cause.

- At first, you may experience lower back discomfort only while sitting for a prolonged period, or on standing up after sitting down. In this case, the pain is caused by the overstretching of soft tissues, and it takes only a few seconds for the tissues to recover. At this stage, the pain exists only for a short time.

- At a later stage, you will find that on standing up you have increased pain, and you must walk carefully for a short distance before you can straighten up fully. Now it is likely that some distortion has occurred in one of the lumbar discs: prolonged sitting has led to minor distortion of a disc, and the disc needs a few minutes to recover.

- Eventually, you may reach the stage where you frequently experience sharp or agonizing pain on standing and you are unable to straighten up even after walking carefully. If this is the case, there is a major distortion of the affected disc, which cannot regain its normal shape quickly enough to allow pain-free movement. Instead, whenever a movement is attempted, the disc bulge increases the strain on the surrounding tissues, which are already overstretched. In addition, the disc bulge may pinch the sciatic nerve, which may cause pain and other symptoms in the leg.

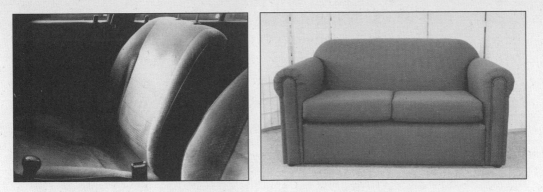

Figure 4.5 *Poorly designed seating*

Environmental Factors

We can blame ourselves for a lot, but if you would prefer to also blame others, this is your opportunity. Designers are out to get you! The design of seating—whether found in transportation, business settings, or the home—is focused more on sales than posture. More specifically, the design seems focused on appearance and an immediate sense of physical comfort, even if in the long run pain and stiffness and even injury is the result.

Seating design contributes to our poor postural habits. Chairs rarely give adequate support to the lower back. Unless you make a conscious effort to sit correctly, you are more or less forced to sit badly (Figs. 4.5).

Ideally, the backs of all chairs would provide a lumbar support so that the lordosis, which is naturally present in standing, is also

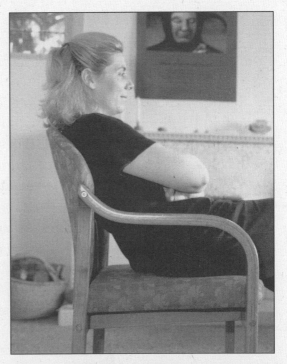

Figure 4.5 *Poor sitting posture*

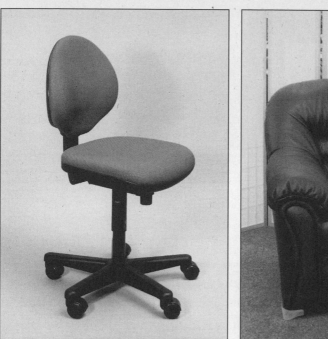

Figure 4.6
Well-designed typist or secretarial chair

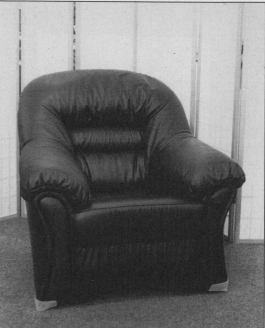

Figure 4.6
Well-designed lounge chair

maintained while sitting (Figs. 4.6). But rarely do seat designers include this support.

Equally important, furniture in offices and factories should be adapted to individual requirements. For example, if you are a desk worker, you must make sure that the seat of your chair has the correct height. This means that as you sit, your feet should rest flat on the floor and your thighs should remain horizontal without your having to press on the seat.

The desk itself must also be the correct height. If the surface you lean on is too low, you will slouch forward and lose the lordosis. If the desk surface is too low, raise the desk by using wooden blocks.

Finally, armrests must be positioned in such a way that, when you use them, your shoulders are neither raised nor lowered too much. Your shoulders are at the wrong height if you feel discomfort in them after 10 to 20 minutes.

Armrests also should allow your chair to be pulled under your desk so that you can sit with your stomach held gently against the front of the desk.

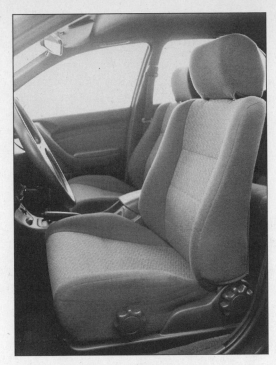

Figure 4.7   *The McKenzie seat*

This will prevent you from leaning over and losing the lordosis while you perform desk tasks.

Until furniture designers understand and defer to the requirements of the human frame, we will continue to suffer from their neglect.

Although the poor design of furniture contributes to the development of lower back problems, equal blame must be placed upon the individual who uses a chair improperly. If we do not know how to sit correctly, even the best chairs will not prevent us from slouching. On the other hand, once we have learned the correct concepts, poorly designed chairs will not have such a detrimental effect on our sitting posture.

Several years ago, the Toyota Motor Corporation in New Zealand asked the McKenzie Institute International to provide expertise to assist the company in the design of new seats for a variety of its vehicles sold in that country. From this cooperative venture has emerged a seat with outstanding qualities. It combines spinal support and driver stability (Fig. 4.7). The seat has met with universal consumer approval, especially when used for extended trips.

Similarly, the McKenzie Institute recently has become involved in the design of furniture for relaxing in the home. It is a goal of the Institute that well-designed home furniture be widely available and affordable.

Sitting Correctly for Long Periods

If you have pain resulting from factors other than just poor posture, you may need to do more than correct your posture. You may need to perform special exercises. In this chapter, I am describing only the exercises required to reduce postural stress and to obtain postural correction. In later chapters, you will find exercises for relief of pain and increase of function in both the back and the neck.

In order to avoid the development of lower back pain due to prolonged poor sitting, it is necessary that you (1) sit correctly and (2) interrupt prolonged sitting at regular intervals.

Correcting the Sitting Posture

From now on, you must pay a lot of attention to your sitting posture. I know this will strike some of you as bad news, or even unnecessary news. The fact is, however, that you can get used to paying more attention to your sitting posture—used to it in such a way that it does not interfere with your life.

Further, the fact is that if you don't take the fairly minimal trouble to correct your sitting posture, you may pay a price far more costly than a relatively simple change in behavior: you may develop back pain that is severe or even disabling, and you may develop the irreversible bent-over posture associated with the elderly.

You may have had the habit of sitting slouched for many years without lower back pain, but once you have developed lower back pain problems, you must no longer sit in the old way. The slouched posture will only perpetuate the overstretching and distortion of the joints.

In order to sit correctly, you must first learn *how to form a lordosis* in the lower back while sitting. Therefore, you must become fully practiced in what I call the *slouch-overcorrect procedure*. Once you have achieved this, you must learn *how to maintain a lordosis* in the lower back while sitting for long periods.

How to Form a Lordosis

You must sit on a stool of chair-height. If a stool is unavailable, the edge of a chair will do. Once seated, allow yourself to slouch completely (Fig. 4.8). Now you are ready to commence the *slouch-overcorrect procedure*.

Relax for a few seconds in the slouched position. Then draw yourself up and accentuate the lordosis as far as possible (Fig. 4.9). This is the extreme of the good sitting position. Hold yourself in this position for a few seconds.

Now return to the fully relaxed position (Fig. 4.8).

Do these movements as you *slowly* think or say the words, "pressure on, pressure off." Remain in the first position during "pressure on," the second position during "pressure off." Combining the words

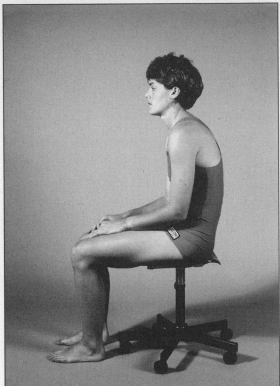

Figure 4.8
Extreme of slouched sitting position

with the movements helps you to hold each position for the right amount of time and to establish a rhythm. The technique of slowly thinking or speaking the words "pressure on, pressure off" can be used with all the McKenzie exercises for the back and neck that involve multiple movements.

In the exercise to form a lordosis, the movement from the slouched position to the upright position should be done in such

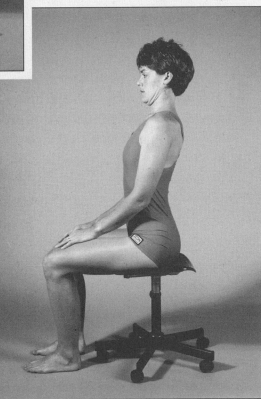

Figure 4.9
Accentuating the lordosis

Case History: Nursing Herself Back to Health

Greta, a 41-year-old nurse, works on a surgical floor at a hospital in Indiana. Her doctor diagnosed her with lumbar radiculitis, meaning she had inflammation of a lumbar nerve root. She had lower back pain as well as leg pain going all the way to her heel. Greta had these symptoms for six months and they were getting worse. She had suffered no injury and had no idea why she had back pain.

The symptoms had begun in her left buttock. Her lower back pain was constant and her leg symptoms intermittent. She had limited range of motion in the back. She was unable to sit for long periods and unable to sleep through the night.

Using McKenzie postural techniques, including the use of a lumbar roll and the "slouch-overcorrect" exercise, Greta was able to sit more comfortably and for longer periods. She also benefitted from Back Exercise 3, Extension in Lying. This greatly reduced her leg symptoms.

A week after starting with the McKenzie Method, Greta's symptoms had centralized, so that they were only in the left buttock. That is, her leg pain was completely gone. She was able to sleep through the night. She had improved range of motion in the lumbar spine.

About 10 days later, she progressed to Flexion in Lying (Back Exercise 5) but kept up with Back Exercise 3 as well. A week later, Greta had no symptoms and full range of motion. She progressed to Flexion in Standing (Back Exercise 7) instead of in lying down, and kept up with Extension in Lying. She remains pain-free.

a way that you move rhythmically from the extreme of the bad to the extreme of the good sitting posture.

Perform the exercise 10 or 15 times per session. Repeat the sessions three times per day, preferably once in the morning, once around noon, and once in the evening. In addition, do the exercise whenever pain arises as a result of sitting poorly. Each time you repeat the cycle of movements (slouch-upright-slouch), be sure the movements are performed to the maximum possible degree, particularly in the upright position.

Farragut Branch Library

777-1750

user ID:40554000064729

title:Brimstone / Douglas Prest
author:Preston, Douglas J.
item id:50551022457a13
due:11/29/2004,23:59

title:Thr3e / Ted Dekker
author:Dekker, Ted, 1962-
item id:50551100027367
due:11/29/2004,23:59

Thank you for visiting the
Knox County Public Library System

Review your account on the web at
www.knoxlib.org

Maintaining the Lordosis

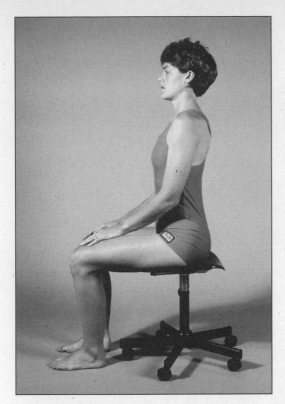

Figure 4.10 *Extreme of good sitting position: less lordosis strain creates correct sitting posture.*

You have just learned how to find the *extreme of the good sitting posture.* It is not possible to sit in this way for long periods, because it causes considerable strain and, if maintained for excessive periods, might actually cause pain. To sit comfortably and correctly, you must sit in a way that is not as upright as the position of extreme good posture. To find the correct position, you must first sit with your lower back in extreme lordosis (Fig. 4.9) and then release the last 10 percent of the lordosis strain. At the same time, take care to ensure that you do not allow the lower back to flatten (Fig. 4.10).

Now you have reached the correct sitting posture, which can be maintained for any length of time. When sitting like this, you maintain the lordosis of the lower back with your own muscular effort. It requires constant attention and constant effort, and you cannot fully relax. And whenever you sit on a seat without a back, you must sit in this way.

The Lumbar Roll

Relatively few chairs' seat backs provide adequate support for the lower back. For this reason, for people with ongoing back problems, a portable lumbar roll is essential equipment. When sitting on a seat that has a back, you will find that a lumbar roll will facilitate the maintenance of a correct lordosis and correct posture.

A lumbar roll (Fig. 4.11) is a fat, cylindrical-shaped support made mostly of foam rubber that is designed specifically for the lower back. Without this

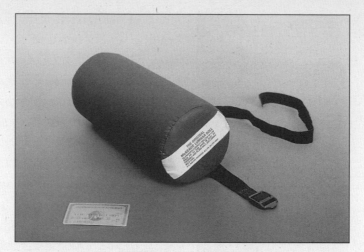

Figure 4.11 Lumbar roll

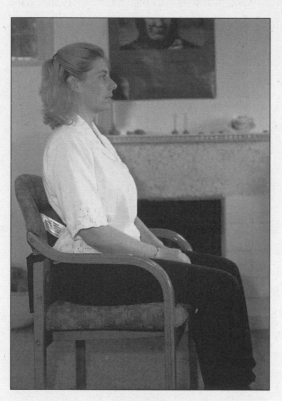

Figure 4.12
Use of lumbar roll to correct poor chair design

support, the lower back will slouch whenever you are distracted or stop concentrating on anything other than holding the lordosis actively with your own muscles. For instance, if you must focus on talking, reading, writing, watching TV, or driving your car, chances are you will lose the lordosis and slouch into bad posture—unless you use a lumbar roll. You may be concentrating on being a brilliant conversationalist, but your lumbar roll is a faithful little fellow, and he's focused on one thing: maintaining your lordosis.

To avoid the slouching that ordinarily would occur as you concentrate on something other than your lordosis and your posture, you must place a lumbar roll in the

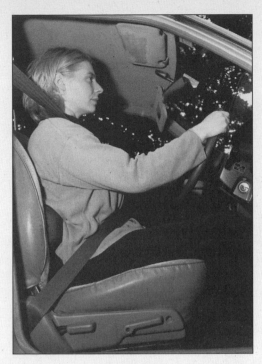

Figure 4.13
Use of lumbar roll to correct poor car seat design

small of your back at the level of your beltline whenever you sit in a standard chair (Fig. 4.12), a car (Fig. 4.13), or an office chair (Figs. 4.14a and 4.14b).

You may purchase a lumbar roll specifically made for the above purpose from the authorized firm listed in Appendix B of this book. You will need to provide your waist measurement and your weight.

The lumbar roll should be no more than four to five inches (about 10–13 centimeters) in diameter before being compressed. It should be filled with foam rubber of moderate density so that when compressed its diameter reduces to about 1.5 inches (about four centimeters).

A regular seat-back cushion does not serve the same purpose as a lumbar roll because it is the wrong shape and does not provide adequate pressure at the key level of the lower back. Do not rely on a regular cushion for long-term use, but it may be of some assistance in an emergency. Also inappropriate for the long-term but of possible value in a pinch is a rolled-up bath towel or beach towel or even a roll of paper towels.

The first aim of this part of the program is to restore the correct posture. The second goal is to maintain it. It may take up to a week to master this fully. *As a rule, pain that is due to bad posture will decrease as your sitting posture improves,* and once you maintain the correct posture, you will have no pain at all. In the first few weeks, if you allow yourself to slouch while sitting, the pain will readily come back. Eventually, though, you will remain completely pain-free even when you forget your posture. Even so, you should never again allow yourself to sit in a slouched position for long periods.

The first few times you use these procedures to correct your sitting posture, you will experience some new pains. These will be different from

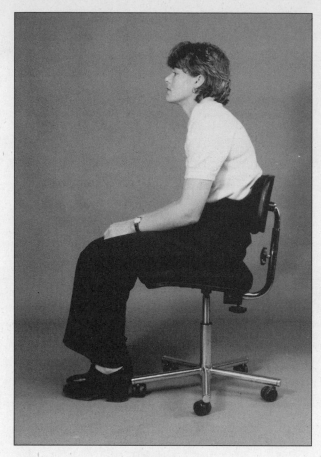

Figure 4.14a
Poor office chair design uncorrected

your original pain, and you may feel them in new places. New pains are the result of performing new exercises and of maintaining new positions. They should be expected, and they will wear off in a few days—*if* you continue to correct your posture on a regular basis. Once you have become used to sitting correctly, you will *enjoy* it. And soon you will notice the reduction or absence of pain and you simply will sit with more comfort. On the other hand, if you slouch, pain can return.

At first, many patients who have become used to sitting correctly do not even notice their symptoms have gone away. Only later does the patient realize that his or her back has become so pain-free that he or she is no longer thinking about it. Once you are used to sitting with the correct posture, you will automatically choose chairs that allow you to sit correctly.

RULE: When sitting for long periods, you must sit correctly: with the lower back in moderate lordosis. Whenever your seat has a back, you must use a lumbar roll to support your lower back.

In 1988, the McKenzie Institute commissioned a study to examine the effects of sitting with and without a lumbar roll. One group used the roll, one group didn't. Those using the roll were required to use it at home, at the office, and when driving. The results showed conclusively that the patients using a lumbar roll whenever sitting experienced much less pain than those not using the roll.

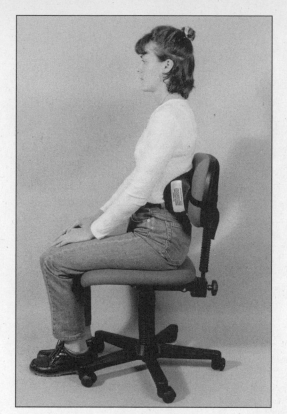

Figure 4.14b
Poor office chair design corrected by lumbar roll

Regularly Interrupting Prolonged Sitting

Traveling for long distances by car, bus, or plane may cause a gradual and progressive attack of lower back pain or may aggravate existing problems. This is the case especially when you sit in a cramped seat and do not take regular breaks that would permit you to restore your lordosis. After an uninterrupted car ride of even a few hours, nearly everyone will notice some stiffness or discomfort in the lower back. If you already have back problems, such a journey may be a risky experience for you. If you are the driver, the risk is even greater than if you are a passenger.

In order to minimize the risks of prolonged sitting, you must interrupt sitting at regular intervals and *before pain starts*. For example, during long car trips, once an hour you should stop the car, get out, bend backward five or six times (see Exercise 4 in the next chapter), and then walk around for a few minutes. This will reduce the pressure within the discs and will relieve the stresses on the surrounding tissues.

As long as airlines continue to provide seating seemingly calculated to damage the human spine, you should take action when traveling on planes

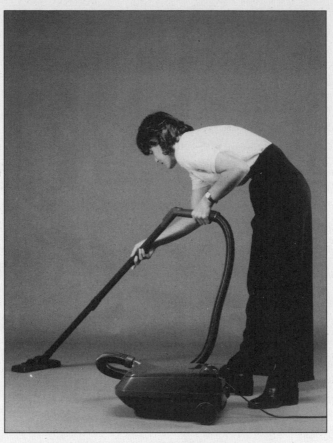

Figure 4.15 *Vacuuming usually involves bending.*

as well. When flying long distances, regularly stand up and walk up and down an aisle of the plane. Not only is this important for your back, but it also stimulates circulation in the legs.

Taking breaks during travel, whether in a car or on a plane, will significantly reduce the risk of another episode of back pain.

RULE: When you sit for prolonged periods, regular interruption of the sitting posture is essential to prevent the onset of pain. You can interrupt this posture by standing upright, bending backward five or six times, and walking about for a few minutes. (See Exercise 4.)

Case History: Furniture Factory

Isaac, 48, is the owner of a furniture factory in Pennsylvania. He himself is one of the furniture makers. He had episodic pain in the right lower back. This resulted from an injury at work suffered while bending over and rotating to the left. He subsequently felt pain when bending, lifting, and sitting.

He had seen a chiropractor, but with little effect. He had been taking the prescription drug Percoset and the over-the-counter medication Aleve.

With the McKenzie Method, he learned to sit correctly at work and while driving and also improved his posture when standing. He also used Back Exercise 3, Extension in Lying, and Back Exercise 4, Extension in Standing. Within two days, his pain was gone. He remained symptom-free.

---

2. WORKING IN STOOPED POSITIONS

Stooped positions often result in back pain. When you stand with your back straight, the stresses on the discs and ligaments of your lower back are considerably lower than when you stand with your back bent forward. Many activities around the home may ordinarily involve bending, for example gardening, vacuuming, and making a bed (Fig. 4.15). Occupations requiring prolonged stooped posture are abundant: assembly-line worker, farmworker, bricklayer, electrician, plumber, carpenter, surgeon, nurse. The list goes on and on. People in all of these occupations are in most cases required to bend forward for prolonged periods every day (Fig. 4.16). While working with a stooped posture, you are most likely to experience back problems in the first four or five hours of the day.

In order to minimize the risks involved in prolonged forward bending, interrupt the stooped position at regular intervals. And it is important that you interrupt it *before pain starts*. Stand upright and bend backward five or six times (see Exercise 4). This is especially important if you already have developed lower back problems by working in a stooped position. Regular interruption of the stooped position will correct any distortion that may

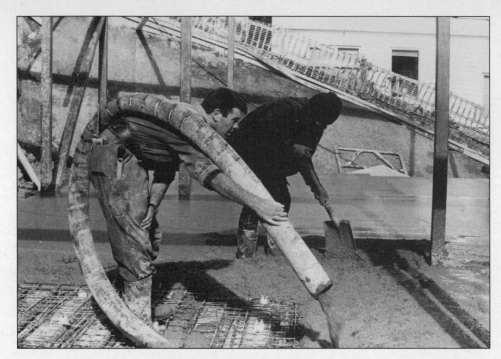

Figure 4.16   *Prolonged stooped position*

have occurred in the discs and will relieve the stresses on the surrounding tissues.

When this interruption occurs before pain starts, it usually prevents the development of significant lower back pain. *Remember: you are especially at risk in the first half of your day,* so make sure you pay attention to your posture during this period.

RULE: When working in a stooped position, you must regularly interrupt bent posture in order to prevent the onset of pain. You can do this by standing upright and bending backward five or six times. (See Exercise 4.)

3. LIFTING

Lifting an object with your back rounded (Fig. 4.17) raises the pressure in your discs to a much higher level than if you were to lift the same object with your body upright and with your lordosis present. Research has borne this out. Just as back problems associated with stooped positions seem to occur very frequently in the first four or five hours of the day (because the discs take up fluid while we rest at night), the same is true with lifting. This is the case especially if you lift repeatedly and frequently. If you use an incorrect technique while lifting a heavy object, you may cause damage and pain, and the pain may be not only sudden but severe.

In order to minimize the risks involved in lifting, always use the correct lifting technique (Figs. 4.17a–e). *Immediately before and after lifting,* stand upright and bend backward five or six times. You should do this especially when a single heavy lift is involved. If you must lift many objects, one after another, frequently interrupt the lifting and repeat the bending backward exercise just described. By standing upright and bending backward before lifting, you ensure that, as you begin the lift, there is no distortion already present in the joints of the lower back. This is particularly important if, immediately before you start lifting, you have been in a stooped position or have been sitting for a long period.

For example, many truck drivers drive for hours and hours and then are called upon to remove heavy objects from the back of their truck. A more common example comes when you take a car trip, sit in the car for several hours before

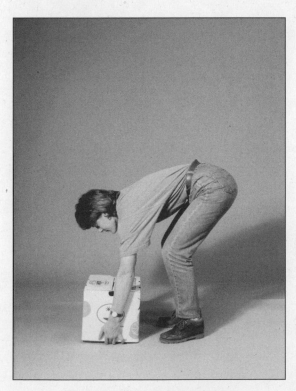

Figure 4.17 *Poor lifting technique*

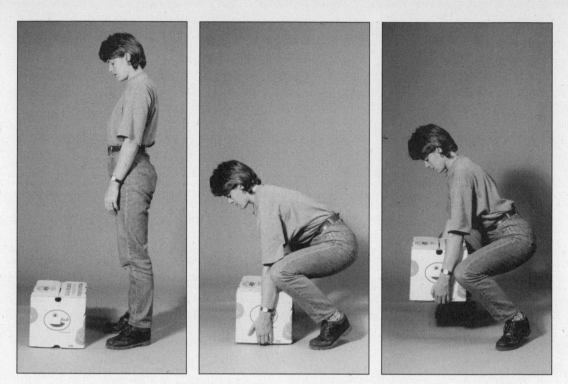

Figures 4.17a–4.17c Correct lifting technique

stopping, arrive at your destination, and remove heavy objects from the trunk. Whether you're a truck driver or a car passenger, when you've been on the road for a long time, take a moment before lifting. Stand upright and bend backward a few times before and after lifting. By doing so, you will correct any distortion that may have developed in the joints as a result of sitting.

If you are suffering from lower back pain right now, and especially if your pain has been caused by lifting, it is best to completely avoid lifting for a few weeks. This will permit damaged tissues to heal. If it is not possible to avoid lifting, you must at all times use the correct lifting technique and avoid lifting objects that are awkward to handle or are heavier than 30 pounds (about 15 kilograms).

Once you have developed recurrent lower back problems, you should never again handle awkward or heavy objects by yourself. This is true even if you are completely free of pain. In addition, you should become familiar with the correct lifting technique. After some practice with this technique, lifting correctly will become a habit.

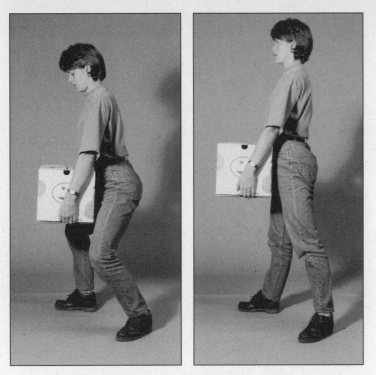

Figures 4.17d–4.17e   *Correct lifting technique*

Correct Lifting Technique

Throughout a lift, you must attempt to retain the lordosis in your lower back (Figs. 4.17a–e). You make the lift by straightening your legs. Avoid using the back as a crane (Fig. 4.17).

Correct lifting technique involves the following:

- Stand close to the load. Have a firm footing and a wide stance.

- Exaggerate the lordosis.

- As you descend to approach the load, bend your knees and keep your back straight.

- Get a secure grip and hold the load as close to your body as possible.

Case History: Getting a Lift

Florence is a 58-year-old cleaning lady who works at a physician's office and who also baby-sits her grandchildren. She lives in Florida. She had distressing lower back pain for two and a half weeks, and had experienced lower back pain off and on for five years. The new episode began when she bent over in her cleaning work. Her pain got worse when she bent, lifted, sat, lay on either side, or walked almost any distance. She was also worse in the morning. Her sitting posture was only fair, and she had pain after sitting for long periods.

Exercise 3, Extension in Lying, reduced her pain, but only during the exercise. She began doing Exercise 3 five times a day and began using a lumbar roll when sitting. Six days later, her back pain had decreased, and she could walk greater distances before the onset of pain.

She learned to improve her posture through the slouch-overcorrect procedure, and she added this to her exercise program, doing it two to three times a day.

Still, bending and lifting at work continued to bother her. She learned to lift properly, not by bending over but rather by maintaining the lordosis in her lumbar spine and using her quadriceps (upper leg) muscles to lift.

She began to do Exercise 4, Extension in Standing, throughout her workday, especially after bending. With the use of the lumbar roll, she found she could sit without pain for longer periods than before.

She began Exercise 5, Flexion in Lying. It caused her no symptoms and no reduction in her ability to extend her spine. She did this exercise two to three times a day, followed by Exercise 3, Extension in Lying. Two weeks after beginning to use these two exercises, she was pain-free and able to resume all her previous activities.

- Lean back to stay in balance, and lift the load by straightening the knees.

- Make the lift with a steady motion. Don't jerk.

- Once you have become upright and you need to turn the weight, turn it by shifting your feet, not by twisting your lower back.

RULE: When lifting, use the correct lifting technique. In addition, immediately before and after each heavy single lift, stand upright and bend backward five or six times. When you lift repeatedly, perform the same exercise at regular intervals.

4. RELAXING AFTER VIGOROUS ACTIVITY

Over the years I have heard many people complain that they develop back pain after engaging in activities such as gardening, laying concrete, or even running. It is easy, even logical, to attribute the pain to the activity. After all, one has followed the other. In many cases, one has followed the other repeatedly: every time the person gardens, he or she has a sore lower back afterward. In fact, however, very often it is not the strenuous physical activity that is the culprit.

Very often, following such an activity, we sit and relax. We may collapse into a slouched position in a chair. We may sit on the grass, bent over at the waist. We may stand, out of breath, bent forward at the waist, supporting our upper body by placing our hands on our knees. After a while we feel pain, and we automatically blame the activity that we have just completed.

Instead, we should consider the likelihood that the pain has begun as a result of the posture we have adopted *since the exercise.* If the activity itself had been responsible for the pain, we would have felt some discomfort or pain during the activity. This would have been due to overstretching or injury occurring during the activity. If we had hurt ourselves during exercise, pain would not likely have arisen significantly after the activity (often, pain following exercise takes an hour or so to arise). Rather, it would have occurred immediately, during the activity.

After activity, the joints of the spine undergo a loosening process. If, after exercise, we place the back in an unsupported position for long periods, distortion within the joint readily occurs. This is true whether we sit in a slouched position or whether we stand, bending forward with our hands on our knees. *Thoroughly exercised joints of the spine distort easily if the spine is placed in a slouched position for long periods.* For more on how pain following an activity often is not caused by the activity itself, see Chapter 8's discussion of sports-related injuries.

> RULE: After vigorous activity, restore and exaggerate the lordosis by standing upright and bending backward five or six times. When you sit down to rest, maintain the lordosis and use a lumbar roll in order to avoid slouching.

5. PROLONGED STANDING

Some people get lower back pain every time they stand in one place for a long time. The same thing happens when we sit for long periods. In either situation, the muscles that support us tire and relax, allowing us to slouch. When we stand in a relaxed manner, however, the lordosis *becomes excessive* and the lower back hangs in an extreme position.

This position is exactly opposite to that adopted by the spine when we sit in a slouch. It is not possible to stand in this relaxed way for long periods, because the excessive lordosis is a position of strain. If your lower back pain occurs during long periods of standing, you will find relief by correcting your standing posture.

> RULE: When standing for long periods, you must stand correctly. Stand tall, and do so frequently. Don't allow your back to sag into extreme lordosis.

Correcting the Standing Posture

To stand correctly, you must hold your lower back in a position of reduced lordosis. To find this position, first you must stand relaxed. Allow the chest to sag and the abdomen to protrude slightly. This will place the lower lumbar joints in an extreme lordosis.

Next, reduce lordosis by standing as tall as you can. Lift the chest up, pull in your stomach, and tighten your buttocks (Fig. 4.18).

You have now reached the correct standing posture. When standing like this, you reduce the lordosis through your own muscular effort.

To begin with, you will find it difficult to hold this position, but with practice you can learn to stand in the new position for long periods without discomfort.

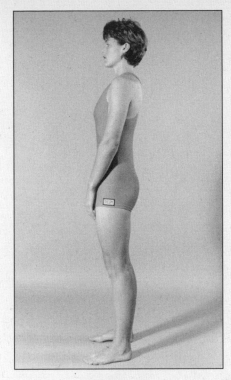

Figure 4.18
Correct standing posture

6. LYING DOWN AND RESTING

Some people have lower back pain when they lie resting in certain positions. A relative few have lower back pain only when they lie down. Many people with lower back pain feel worse when they are lying down, and they dread the thought of another night with more back pain and less sleep.

If you have lower back pain only when you are lying down, or if you regularly awake in the morning with a stiff and painful lower back that was not painful the night before, one of two things is probably wrong. Either there is something wrong with the surface on which you are lying, or there is something wrong with the position in which you sleep (Fig. 4.19).

It is a comparatively easy task to correct the surface on which you are lying, but it is rather difficult to influence the position you adopt while sleeping. Once you are asleep, you may frequently change your position or "toss and turn." Unless a certain position causes so much discomfort that it wakes you up, you will have no idea of the various positions you assume while sleeping.

Many people with back problems are told never to lie facedown while in bed. This can indeed make it difficult to recover from an injury to the

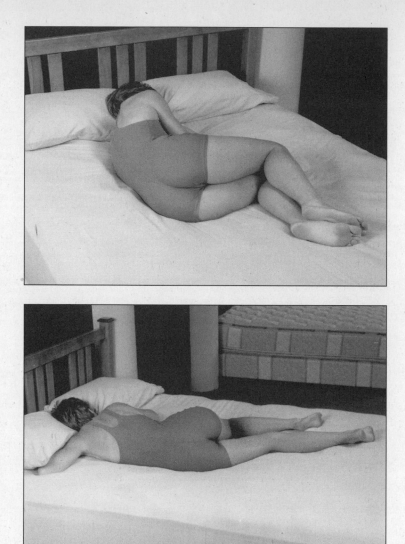

Figure 4.19 *Poor lying position*

neck, but there is no evidence whatsoever to suggest that this is harmful to the back. On the contrary, it may well be that your back will stop being painful if you sleep in the facedown position.

If you have not already discovered the effects of lying facedown, you should experiment. Next time you have back pain while lying down, see what effect lying facedown has on your problem. The results will vary from person to person. Certainly there are some lower-back problems that are aggravated by lying facedown. And if you have sciatica, lying facedown is nearly always impossible. But for many back sufferers, lying facedown will bring relief.

Case History: Numbness and Tingling

Rose, 76, from Florida, is a retiree whose physician had diagnosed her with lumbar radiculitis (inflammation of a lumbar nerve root). For two months, she'd had lower back pain as well as numbness and tingling in the right leg and foot. Her symptoms came and went but were most often provoked by sitting. Her pain interrupted her sleep.

Extension in Lying (Back Exercise 3) reduced Rose's symptoms in the right leg and foot.

Five days later she had less numbness and tingling in the foot but more of each in the thigh. Using a lumbar roll while sitting had reduced the symptoms in the foot. Per the McKenzie Method, she was sleeping on her stomach, and this further reduced the foot problems.

Two days later Rose was able to sit for longer periods and was sleeping much better, and her leg symptoms had declined dramatically. Back Exercise 3 remained the key one for her.

Four days later, she was sleeping through the night and her foot symptoms were better still. She used the "slouch-overcorrect" posture exercise without difficulty and it helped to improve her posture.

Two days later Rose could easily tolerate Flexion in Lying (Back Exercise 5). Five days after that, she was symptom-free. She progressed to Flexion in Standing (Back Exercise 7).

She remained free of pain and had full range of motion.

Correcting the Surface

There are two simple ways in which you may be able to reduce strain on your lower back caused by a faulty lying position:

The first and most important way is to lie with a supportive lumbar roll around your waist. The roll will support your lower back as you rest, and it will prevent the strain that can develop when you lie on your side or back.

You may purchase a lumbar night roll specifically made for this purpose from the firm mentioned in Appendix B of this book. You will need to supply your waist measurement and your weight.

A good temporary alternative is to use a rolled beach towel or bath towel. Fold the towel in half from end to end, then roll it from the side.

Your goal is to create a roll of about three inches (about 7.5 centimeters) in diameter and three feet (about 90 centimeters) in length. Wind the roll around your waist at the level where you normally wear a belt and hold it together in front with a safety pin to ensure that it remains in place. If the towel is not held together properly, the roll may move up or down during your sleep. If the towel has moved to the wrong place, it may actually *increase* your pain during or after sleep.

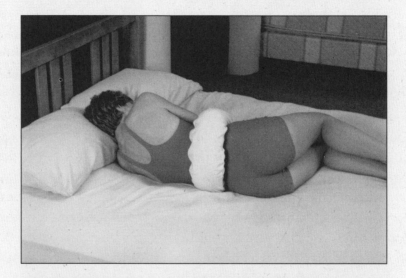

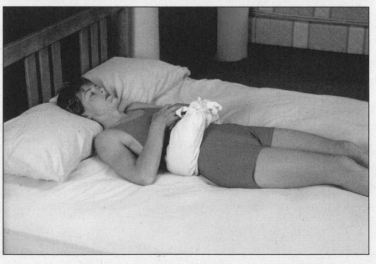

Figure 4.20   *Lying position corrected by lumbar night roll*

The diameter and length given above are merely a guide: lumbar supports need to fulfill individual requirements, and each person must experiment for himself or herself. You can follow the general rule that when you lie on your side, the roll should fill the natural hollow in the body's shape between the pelvis and the rib cage. The other general rule is that when you lie on your back, the roll should support the lower back, placing it in moderate lordosis (Fig. 4.20).

The second way to reduce strain on your lower back is to ensure that your mattress does not sag. The mattress itself should not be too hard. In fact, a soft mattress can be extremely comfortable, provided it is placed on a firm support.

To ensure that your mattress is supported on a firm, hard surface, it is best to experiment by placing it on the floor. Spend three to four nights sleeping with the mattress supported in this manner; this will allow you to determine if poor support for your mattress is the source of your back pain.

Avoid a bed with a wire base. (Commonly used in the fifties and sixties, this is a base or frame with wires stretched across it and adjusted with bolts.) Use a firm base; a box spring may be used if it is firm and does not sag. Another example of a firm base would be the solid wood base found in a bed frame made to support a mattress alone, as opposed to a metal frame designed to support a box spring and mattress. If a solid base is not readily available, the effects of a soft box spring can be reduced by inserting slats or a bed board—a rigid piece of plywood—between the box spring and mattress.

The mattress itself may be either of the most common types: innerspring or foam rubber.

If you have tried these suggestions without benefit, consult a health care provider trained in the treatment of lower back pain. Members and associates of the McKenzie Institute are well versed in the management of problems relating to lying and resting. It may be that you need special advice regarding the surface on which you lie or the posture you assume while you sleep. It may also be that you need special treatment for your lower back problems.

7. COUGHING AND SNEEZING

Coughing and sneezing while you are bent forward or sitting may cause a sudden attack of lower back pain, or may aggravate existing back pain. If you sense the need to cough or sneeze, try to stand upright and bend backward before coughing or sneezing, so that your lower back is hollow—in lordosis—at the moment the cough or sneeze comes. Should you not be able to stand up, at least lean backward, making the best possible lordosis.

5 The McKenzie Method Exercises for the Back

GENERAL GUIDELINES AND PRECAUTIONS

The McKenzie back exercise program consists of seven exercises. The McKenzie neck exercise program consists of seven different exercises; you will find them in Chapter 12.

Even though there are seven exercises, it is unlikely that in any one exercise session you will need to do more than two. So the exercise program is neither hard nor time-consuming.

The first four back exercises are extension exercises, and the last three are flexion exercises. In regard to the back, extension means bending backward, and flexion means bending forward.

The purpose of the exercises is to eliminate pain and, where possible, to restore normal function—that is, to regain full mobility in the lower back or as much movement as possible under the circumstances. When you are exercising for pain relief, you move to the edge of the pain or just into the pain, then release the pressure and return to the starting position. But when you are exercising in order to regain lost movement or to reduce stiffness, try to attain the maximum amount of movement; to do this, you may have to move well into the pain.

Postural correction and maintenance of the correct posture should always follow the exercises. Even when you no longer have lower back pain, good postural habits are essential to prevent the recurrence of your problems. These habits, therefore, should be followed for the rest of your life.

THE EXERCISES ARE ONLY PART OF THE McKENZIE METHOD

Soon we will get to specific exercises that can give you relief promptly or even immediately. But first, let's discuss the benefits of the exercises in general.

Obviously, the McKenzie exercises eliminate or dramatically reduce pain and stiffness. But the McKenzie Method is much more than exercises. And the exercises are much more than extension: some of them involve the opposite movement, which is called *flexion*.

The McKenzie Method involves instructing back and neck sufferers in how their spine works and how—especially through bad posture in sitting and standing—they are hurting themselves. Consistent with this, it also involves helping people with back or neck pain to correct their daily habits so that they can become pain-free.

A further hallmark of the McKenzie Method is that its exercises typically cause more than relief of pain and stiffness; they also cause a *centralization* of pain or stiffness. When symptoms centralize, they move to the center of the spine, or close to the center, where they are almost always more tolerable than at their more distant locations, even though the pain may increase. Back pain that has radiated down the legs, sometimes as far as the feet, becomes localized in or near the center of the lower back; back pain that is felt mostly on the right or left of the lower back becomes localized closer to its center. This is proof that the exercises are effective for the particular back sufferer, and readers doing the exercises should watch for this encouraging effect.

Health professionals worldwide have confirmed my discovery that centralization is the primary indicator of good progress, shows that the exercises will help, and demonstrates that an expert need not be consulted. In most cases, you can make the same determination yourself: if, after doing the exercises for a while, your pain centralizes, you very likely can treat yourself successfully, without relying on health care providers.

Research has shown that in many instances, centralization is as effective

Case History: Centralization in Texas

Walt is from Texas. He is 54 years old and works as an insurance broker. For two months he had intermittent pain in the central and lower left back. This had come on for no apparent reason. It spread to his left buttock and thigh, and the symptoms were worse when he bent forward, sat, rose to stand, coughed, or sneezed. He felt better when he moved, especially when he walked, and especially later in the day.

He had poor sitting posture and a slight loss of range of motion in lumbar extension. His first McKenzie exercise was Back Exercise 3, Extension in Lying. He moved on to Flexion in Standing (Back Exercise 7), which reduced his pain during the exercise but not after. He also learned the McKenzie techniques of postural correction, especially the "slouch-overcorrect" movements.

Within two days, Walt's back pain had centralized but was more intense. Overall, however, this was a good sign, a sign that he could treat himself successfully with the McKenzie exercises. He continued with Exercise 3, about every two hours during the day. Within two more days, his back pain was gone and his range of motion was complete. With continuation of Exercise 3 and other McKenzie extension exercises, he remained free of symptoms.

as an MRI (magnetic resonance imaging) in determining the nature of a patient's problems. In addition, very recent studies show the McKenzie Method's assessment techniques identify intact discs and demonstrate good progress.

PAIN INTENSITY AND PAIN MOVEMENT
Read This Section Carefully.

The exercises in this book are not designed to strengthen the muscles of your back. We have found that if we can rid you of pain and return you to normal activity, then in the normal course of events your strength will return.

The exercises are designed to correct any distortion or bulging that may have developed in the joints of the lower back. By reducing the distortion or bulging of the intervertebral disc, we can in turn reduce the level of pain that you experience.

The exercises also will identify for you any movements or postures that are likely to increase the distortion in the joints and therefore delay recovery. In turn, your experience with the exercises will enable you to avoid damaging postures and activities in the future.

There are three main effects that you can look for when performing the exercises:

- First, the exercises may cause the symptoms to disappear. This may occur almost immediately or over the course of one to four weeks.

- Second, they may cause an increase or decrease in the intensity of the pain that you experience.

- Third, they may cause the pain to move from where you usually feel it to some other location. In certain cases, the symptoms first will change location, then decrease in intensity, and finally cease altogether.

In summary and addition, pain can improve in many ways:

- It can become less intense.

- It can become less frequent.

- You can sustain activity longer before the pain occurs.

- You can move farther before pain begins.

- Constant pain can be replaced by intermittent pain.

- Pain can centralize. (This not only provides for a more comfortable type of pain but predicts a good outcome through the McKenzie exercises.)

Each one of these improvements is an indication that your condition is improving.

The effects of exercise on the intensity or location of pain can sometimes be very rapid. It is possible to reduce the intensity or change the location of back pain after completing as few as 10 or 12 movements (that is, as few as two repetitions of a session in which an exercise is done five or six times). Sometimes, the pain will completely disappear with just that small amount of effort.

In order to determine whether the exercise program is working effectively for you, it is very important that you observe closely any changes in the intensity or location of your pain. You may notice that as a result of the exercises, the pain, originally felt across the lower back, to one side of the spine, or in one buttock or thigh, moves toward the center of the lower back. In other words, you may notice that your pain *localizes or centralizes.*

Centralization of pain (Fig. 5.0) that occurs as you exercise is a good sign. If your pain moves to the midline of the spine and away from areas where it is usually felt, this means you are exercising correctly and that the McKenzie exercise program is the correct one for you.

The centralization of pain is the single most important guide you have in determining which exercises are correct for your problem. The phenomenon of centralization of pain has now been scientifically validated. Several studies in the United States have demonstrated that if your pain centralizes when you perform the exercises, your chances of rapid and complete recovery are *excellent.*

On the other hand, *avoid activities or positions that cause the pain to "peripheralize"—to move away from the center of the lower back or from the lower back entirely. Also avoid activities and positions that increase any pain in the buttock or leg.*

When first doing the exercises, be cautious and don't hurry. If your lower back pain is of such intensity that you can move around only with difficulty and cannot find a position in which to lie comfortably in bed, you should approach the exercises in an especially cautious and unhurried manner.

When you begin any of the exercises, you may at first experience an increase in pain. *This initial increase of pain is common and can be expected.* As you continue to practice, the pain should quickly diminish, at least to the level you experienced before beginning the exercises. *The reduction of pain, at least to the original level, usually occurs during the first exercise session.* In the first exercise session or a later one, the reduction of pain should be followed by centralization of pain.

Once the pain no longer spreads outward and instead is felt only at the midline, the intensity of pain will decrease rapidly over a period of two to three days. In one to four weeks, your pain should disappear entirely.

If, following an initial increase in pain, the pain continues to increase or spreads to places farther away from the spine, immediately stop exer-

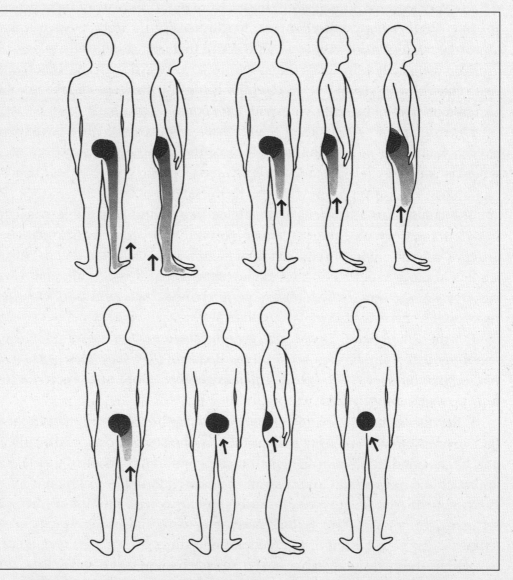

Figure 5.0 *The progressive centralization of pain as a result of the McKenzie exercise program*

cising. Seek advice from a health professional. In other words, do not continue with any of the exercises if your symptoms are much worse immediately after exercising and remain throughout the day. Also stop the exercises if, during exercise, you experience symptoms in the leg below the knee for the first time or if you experience a worsening in symptoms that you already had below the knee.

If your symptoms have been present more or less continuously for many weeks or months, you should not expect to be pain-free in two or three days. The response will be slower than if your symptoms were recent, but if you are doing the correct exercises, it will usually be only a week before improvement begins. If you are lucky, it will be faster than that.

When beginning this exercise program, you should stop any other exercises that you may have been shown by a health professional. You should also temporarily stop any workouts or sports activities. If you want to continue with exercises other than those described in this book, you should wait until your pains have completely subsided. If you are intent on returning to sports before your pain has subsided, you must nonetheless avoid all contact sports. As for non-contact sports, you can gently attempt a return to them; if, after a short trial, your pain is worse, you must discontinue even non-contact sports until your pains have completely subsided.

Once you have started this exercise program, new pains may develop, because you are performing movements your body is not used to. But, provided you continue with the exercises, these pains will wear off in a few days. I always suspect that if my patients have not complained of new pains, they have not been exercising adequately or they have not been putting enough effort into correcting their posture. Both new exercises and new postures *should* cause temporary new pains.

I cannot overstress the importance of doing the exercises precisely as they are described in this book. That is, it is important to do each exercise exactly as it is described and to do the exercises in the order that is set out in this book. The failure to heed even one sentence in the description of an exercise can keep the exercise from being effective. Don't figure that you can save time by glancing at the instructions for a particular exercise or by trying to learn an exercise just by looking at the photographs that accompany it. In this way you may save a minute or two, but may slow your recovery by weeks—not a good bargain.

Similarly, don't skimp. Generally, the exercises should be done six to eight times a day. If you do them once or twice a day, you may gain some benefit, but not nearly what you would gain if you did them as often as prescribed.

RESEARCH SUPPORTS THE METHOD

There are decades of clinical experience and research behind these exercises: how to do them, in what order to do them, how often to do them.

Research findings presented in Adelaide, Australia, in April 2000 are as important as any research ever done on the McKenzie Method. This research was presented to the International Society for the Study of the Lumbar Spine. It reported on a study of patients who had suffered from back pain for an average of 10.4 years. They had seen an average of 2.5 health-care providers before entering the study.

As an abstract of the study says, "this is a dissertation-based investigation of the impact of reading a specific booklet on the LBP [low back pain] and self-treatment behaviour of volunteer chronic symptomatic subjects." These subjects were not treated by doctors, physical therapists, or anybody else. They were treated only by themselves, and the only information they had was a "booklet." In fact, the "booklet" was a detailed description of the McKenzie Method, demonstrating the exercises and posture control found in the book you are reading.

One week after reading the booklet, 86 percent were confident they could treat their own pain effectively. Eighty-five percent said they would use the booklet as a reference and would also use it to "self-treat" in the event of an acute episode and to prevent pain in the future.

Fifty-two percent reported reduced pain in the first week. Once the subjects had used the booklet for nine months, 87 percent were still regularly using the exercises in the booklet and 91 percent were still focusing on good posture.

Most important, at nine months, 82 percent had less back pain and 60 percent were completely free of pain. Ninety-five percent said the booklet was responsible for their improvement.

At the beginning of the study, subjects reported pain that averaged 1.3

on a scale of 4. At nine months, subjects reported pain that averaged only 0.44 on the same scale.

At the start, subjects reported an average of 4.1 episodes of back pain per year. After reading the booklet, they averaged just 1.0 episode per year. (Undermann, B. et al.: "Can an Educational Booklet Change Behavior and Pain in Chronic Low Back Patients?" International Society for the Study of the Lumbar Spine; 2000; Adelaide, Australia.)

These subjects did well because they carefully followed the instructions in the booklet. Similarly, you will do well if you carefully follow the instructions in this book. I want you to benefit as much as possible from the exercises and posture control. Don't get in the way of your own recovery!

BACK EXERCISE 1
Lying Facedown

This is the first McKenzie exercise for the *lower back*. Again, if you are a *neck* patient, you will find the McKenzie exercises for the neck in Chapter 12.

An exercise session is a series of repetitions of one or more exercises. Until you can do one or more of the other McKenzie exercises without acute pain, each time you exercise you must begin with Exercise 1, followed by Exercise 2.

Lie facedown with your arms next to your body. Your arms should be straight but relaxed. Your head should be turned to one side. (See Fig. 5.1.)

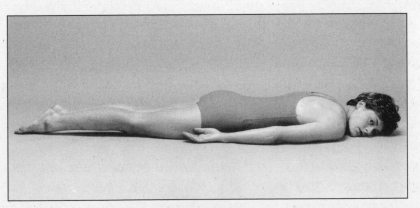

Figure 5.1
Lie facedown with your arms next to your body and your head turned to one side.

Stay in this position, then take a few deep breaths, and then relax completely for two or three minutes. You must make a conscious effort to remove all tension from the muscles in your lower back: without this complete relaxation, there is no chance of eliminating any distortion that may be present in the joint.

Exercise 1 is used mainly in the treatment of acute back pain (back pain that has begun recently and is sharp, as opposed to chronic back pain, which has gone on for a long time and is rather a dull ache). In fact, Exercise 1 is one of the McKenzie Method's *first-aid exercises*. This exercise should be done once at the beginning of each exercise session. Ordinarily, you should do this exercise once per session, but you may feel free to do it more often than that. The exercise sessions should be spread evenly six to eight times throughout the day. This means that you should repeat the sessions about every two hours. In addition, you should lie facedown whenever you are resting.

Exercise 1 is performed in preparation for Exercise 2.

BACK EXERCISE 2
Lying Facedown in Extension

Exercise 2 must be done only after Exercise 1 has been completed. Remain facedown (Fig. 5.2a), in the same position you used in Exercise 1.

Now place your elbows under your shoulders so that you lean on your forearms (Fig. 5.2b). During this exercise (as with Exercise 1), begin by taking a few deep breaths and then allowing the muscles in the lower back to relax completely. Remain in this position for two to three minutes.

Exercise 2 is used mainly in the treatment of acute lower back pain and, like Exercise 1, is one of the *first-aid exercises*. It is also of great benefit for patients with chronic or recurrent problems. Exercise 2 should be done once per exercise session. As with Exercise 1, the sessions should be repeated about every two hours.

If you experience acute, increasing pain when you attempt this exercise, move your elbows farther away from your body, so that your top half is lowered to a point at which your pain is tolerable. Alternatively, you can place a pillow under your chest for a few moments until the pain decreases.

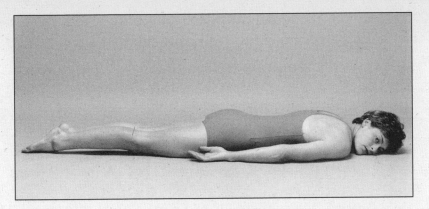

Figure 5.2a Remain facedown.

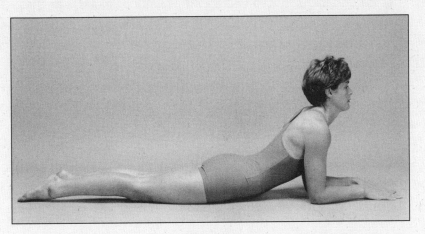

Figure 5.2b
Place your elbows under your shoulders so that you lean on your forearms.

If these efforts are not helpful, there are certain measures you must take before you can continue exercising. These are discussed in the next chapter, under the heading "No Response or Benefit." Go to that section now.

This exercise is performed in preparation for Exercise 3.

BACK EXERCISE 3
Extension in Lying

Before doing this exercise for the first time, start your exercise session with Exercise 1, followed by Exercise 2.

Remain facedown, but with your head forward rather than to the side

Case History: Engineering Her Own Recovery

Helen is a civil engineer, age 52, and lives in upstate New York. She had lower back pain for eight years. The pain was worse when she sat or bent over. She got some relief simply by using a lumbar roll, by walking, and by standing.

Before starting the McKenzie program, Helen had seen numerous physical therapists and a chiropractor, had attended a "back school," and had endured two epidural injections for pain. A doctor had diagnosed degenerative disc disease.

Helen used Back Exercise 3, Extension in Lying. This led to increased extension range without any worsening of pain. Five days after starting the program, her lower back pain had decreased. Helen continued with Back Exercise 3, making a special effort to "sag" as much as possible. Sagging caused pain at the end range of motion, but the pain did not remain when she left the extreme-sag position.

Two days later Helen had full range of motion. She began the "slouch-over-correct" posture exercise without any pain and was able to do Back Exercise 4, Extension in Standing, fully extended.

Five days later, she progressed to Flexion in Lying (Back Exercise 5).

Seventeen days later, Helen had no symptoms at all. Even two weeks later, she had no pain and no limitation in range of motion.

(Fig. 5.3a). Place your hands under your shoulders in the position you would use for a push-up (Fig. 5.3b). Now you are ready to commence Exercise 3.

Straighten your elbows and push the top half of your body—the part from the pelvis on up—up as far as pain permits (Fig. 5.3c). As you do this, it is important that you completely relax the pelvis, hips, and legs. *Keep your pelvis, hips, and legs hanging limp and allow your back to sag*. Your pelvis will naturally move downward.

Once you have maintained this position for a second or two, lower yourself to the starting position. Each time you repeat the cycle of movements in this exercise, try to raise your upper body a little higher, so that by the last repetition of this exercise within a session your back is extended as much as possible and your arms are as straight as possible with your elbows locked (Fig. 5.3d).

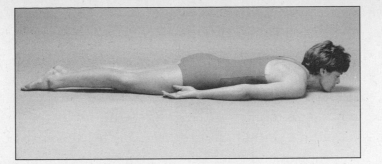

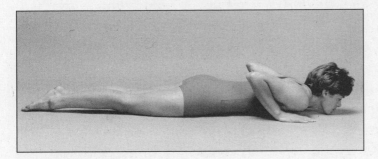

Figure 5.3a
Remain facedown.

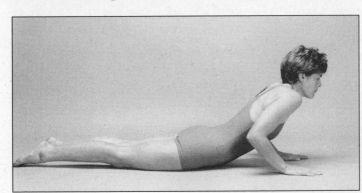

Figure 5.3b   *Place your hands under your shoulders in the push-up position.*

Figure 5.3c   *Straighten your elbows and push the top half of your body up as far as pain permits.*

Figure 5.3d   *At the end of the exercise, your back is extended as much as possible and your arms are as straight as possible.*

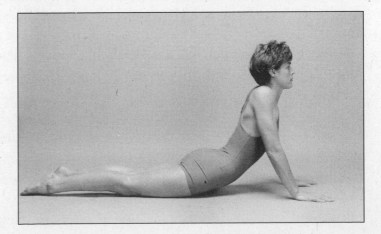

Each time you straighten your arms, remember to hold the sag for a second or two, because this is a key part of the exercise. If you feel your pain is decreasing or centralizing (or both), you may maintain the sag for longer than one or two seconds.

As with all other McKenzie Method back and neck exercises involving multiple movements, remember to slowly think or say the words "pressure on, pressure off," as you do the exercise. This helps you to hold each position just long enough and establishes a rhythm in which to do the exercise.

Exercise 3 is the most useful and effective first-aid procedure in the treatment of acute lower back pain. The exercise can also be used to treat stiffness of the lower back and to prevent lower back pain from recurring once you have fully recovered. When used in the treatment of either pain or stiffness, the exercise should be performed ten times per session. Again, exercise sessions should be spread evenly six to eight times throughout the day.

Should you not respond to Exercise 3 or should you have increasing pain when you attempt this exercise, there are certain measures you must take before you can continue exercising. These are discussed in the next chapter, under the heading "No Response or Benefit." Go to that section now.

Remember that if your pain has *centralized*, it may have *increased* in the middle of your back after it has disappeared from one side or from your leg. This does *not* indicate that you are not responding or benefitting. In fact, this is a good response, and you should continue with the exercises. If the pain has increased but has centralized, you need not read "No Response or Benefit."

BACK EXERCISE 4
Extension in Standing

Stand upright, with your feet slightly apart. Place your hands in the small of your back with the fingers pointing backward (Figs. 5.4a). You are now ready to begin Exercise 4.

Bend your trunk backward at the waist *as far as you can*, using your hands as a fulcrum (Figs. 5.4b). As you do this, it is important that you *keep your knees straight*. Once you have maintained this position for a second or two, return to the starting position. Each time you repeat the cycle of movements in this exercise, try to bend backward a little farther so that by the last repetition your back is extended as far as possible.

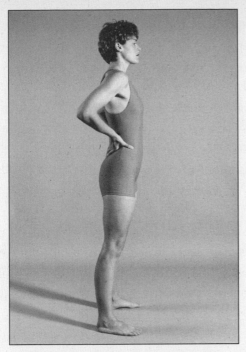

Figure 5.4a *Stand upright, with your feet slightly apart. Place your hands in the small of your back with your fingers pointing backward.*

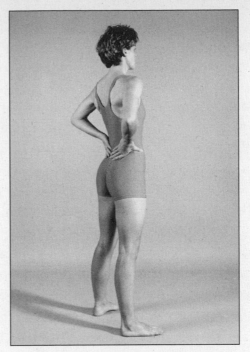

Figure 5.4a *The same position, from a different perspective.*

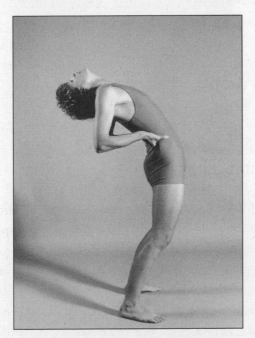

Figure 5.4b *Bend your trunk backward at the waist as far as you can, using your hands as a fulcrum.*

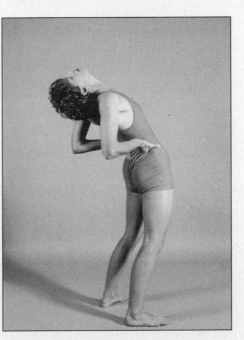

Figure 5.4b *The same position, from a different perspective.*

When you are in acute pain, Exercise 4 may replace Exercise 3 if circumstances prevent you from exercising in the lying position. Nevertheless, this exercise is not as effective as Exercise 3. In the event that you replace Exercise 3 with Exercise 4, do Exercise 4 as often as you would have done Exercise 3, that is, 10 times per session, six to eight sessions a day.

Once you are fully recovered and no longer have lower back pain, Exercise 4 is *your main tool in the prevention of further lower back problems.* As a preventive measure, repeat Exercise 4 every once in a while whenever you find yourself working in a forward-bent position. Perform the exercise *before* the pain appears.

One of the beauties of Exercise 4 is that it can be done without lying down. Therefore, in public or business settings, you can do this exercise more easily than you can perform those that require you to lie down. Still, you should make every effort to find a way to do the lying-down exercises approximately every two hours.

BACK EXERCISE 5
Flexion in Lying

Although some who have heard of the McKenzie Method believe it involves extension and nothing but extension, this is not the case. I have found that for many patients, certain flexion exercises can also be helpful. But especially with the flexion exercises, timing is the key to success. (See later in this chapter; also see Chapter 6, When to Do the Back Exercises.)

Lie on your back with your knees bent and your feet flat on the floor or bed (Fig. 5.5a). You are now ready to begin Exercise 5.

Bring both knees up toward your chest (Fig. 5.5b). Place both hands around your knees and gently but firmly pull your knees as close to your chest as pain permits (Fig. 5.5c). Once you have maintained this position for a second or two, lower the legs and return to the starting position. It is important that you *do not raise your head* as you perform this exercise. It also is important that you *do not straighten your legs as you lower them.*

Each time you repeat the cycle of movements in this exercise, try to pull your knees a little closer to the chest, so that by the last repetition of this exercise you have flexed your back as much as possible.

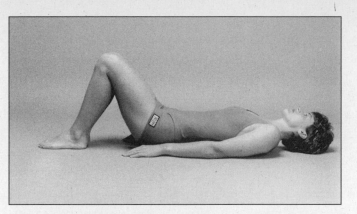

Figure 5.5a   *Lie on your back with your knees bent and your feet flat on the floor or bed.*

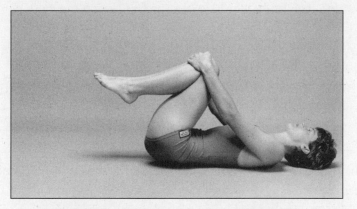

Figure 5.5b   *Bring both knees up toward your chest.*

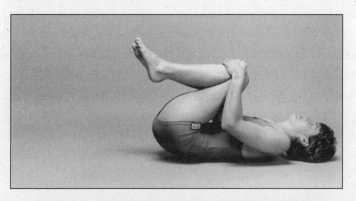

Figure 5.5c   *Place both hands around your knees and gently but firmly pull your knees as close to your chest as pain permits.*

Case History: Garden State

Juan is 64 and manages a plant nursery. He lives in New Jersey. Before beginning the McKenzie program, he had suffered from central lower back pain for three weeks. This appeared after a week during which an employee was out sick and Juan did a lot of stooping as he performed the tasks of the employee. The pain spread to his right calf, and his doctor diagnosed him as having sciatica.

Any activity made his symptoms worse, to the point that he had to lie down to get relief. These activities included sitting, standing, and walking. A non-McKenzie physical therapist had instructed Juan to do exercises that involved lumbar flexion, and these only made his pain more intense.

Juan's posture, though not perfect, was fairly erect, and his range of motion was normal for his age. Though lumbar flexion movements had worsened his pain, he found that the opposite, McKenzie Back Exercise 3, Extension in Lying, eliminated it. He also found it helpful to improve his posture by using the "slouch-overcorrect" method and a lumbar roll.

With the McKenzie program, Juan remained pain-free even during the activities that previously had caused him symptoms.

You can use this exercise to treat stiffness in the lower back that may have developed since your injury began. While damaged tissues may now have healed, they may also have shortened and become less flexible. It is now necessary to restore their elasticity and full function by performing flexion exercises.

Begin these exercises with caution. Do only five or six repetitions per session, and repeat the sessions three or four times a day. As you have probably realized, once your knees are bent in this exercise, you have eliminated the lordosis. Therefore, in order to correct any distortion that may result, *this and all other flexion exercises (that is, Exercise 5, Exercise 6, and Exercise 7) must always be followed immediately by a session of Exercise 3, Extension in Lying.*

BACK EXERCISE 6
Flexion in Sitting

Begin doing Exercise 6 only after you have completed one week of Exercise 5, whether or not Exercise 5 has been successful in reducing your pain or stiffness.

Sit on the edge of a steady chair. Your knees and feet should be well apart. Rest your hands on your legs (Fig. 5.6a). Now you are ready to begin Exercise 6.

Bend your trunk forward and grasp your ankles or touch the floor with your hands (Fig. 5.6b). Return immediately to the starting position. Each time you repeat the cycle of movements in this exercise, try to bend down a little farther so that by the last repetition of this exercise you have flexed your back as much as possible and your head is as close as possible to the floor.

This exercise can be made more effective by holding onto your ankles with your hands and pulling yourself down farther (Figs. 5.6c and 5.6d).

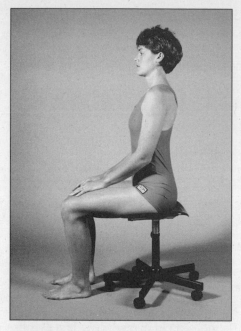

Figure 5.6a *Sit on the edge of a steady chair with your knees and feet well apart and rest your hands on your legs.*

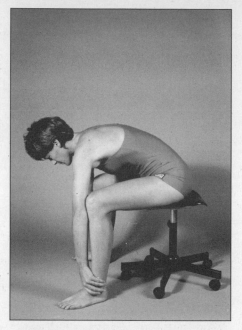

Figure 5.6b *Bend your trunk forward and grasp your ankles or touch the floor with your hands.*

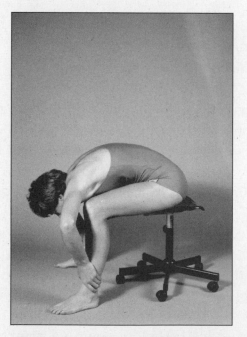

Figure 5.6c *Hold onto your ankles and pull yourself down farther.*

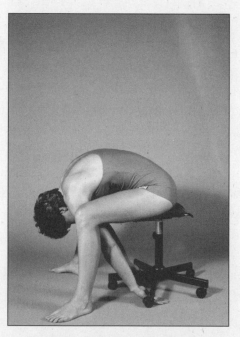

Figure 5.6d *Or even farther.*

You must do only five or six repetitions of Exercise 6 per session. Sessions are to be repeated three to four times a day. *Exercise 6 must always be followed immediately by Exercise 3.*

BACK EXERCISE 7
Flexion in Standing

Begin doing Exercise 7 only after you have completed two weeks of Exercise 6, whether or not Exercise 6 has been successful in reducing your pain or stiffness.

Stand upright, with your feet well apart. Allow your arms to hang loosely by your side (Fig. 5.7a). You are now ready to begin Exercise 7.

Bend forward and run your fingers down your legs as far as you can comfortably reach (Fig. 5.7b). Return immediately to the upright standing

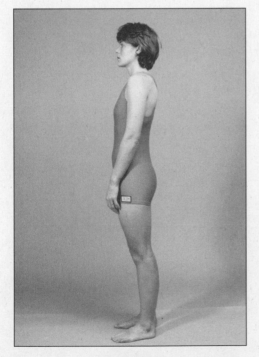

Figure 5.7a
Stand upright with your feet well apart and allow your arms to hang loosely by your side.

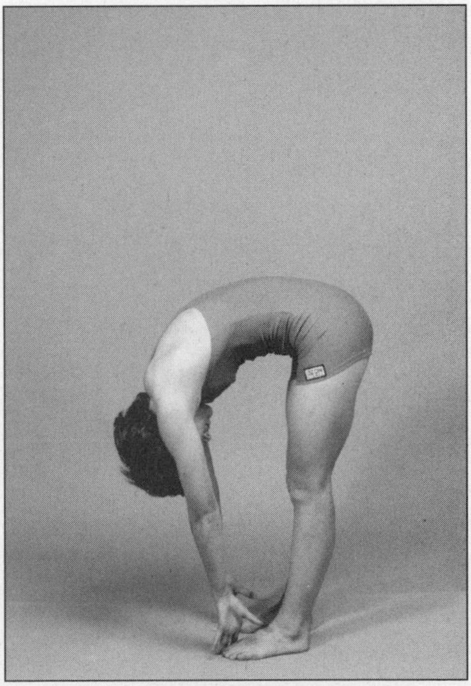

Figure 5.7b
Bend forward and run your fingers down your legs as far as you can comfortably reach.

position. Each time you repeat the cycle of movements in this exercise, try to bend down a little farther so that by the last repetition of this exercise within a session you have flexed your back as much as possible and your fingertips are as close as possible to the floor.

You must do only five or six repetitions of Exercise 7 per session. Sessions are to be repeated once or twice a day. *Exercise 7 must always be followed immediately by Exercise 3.*

For three months after you have become pain-free, Exercise 7 must never be performed in the first four hours of your day.

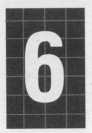

6

When to Do
the Back Exercises

You probably have experienced several acute or severe episodes of back pain in the past. You probably already know that the pain will decrease in time. Still, you may never have been completely free of pain. (Chronic patients can find special hope in the recent research, mentioned earlier, that studied people who had had back pain for 10 years. After nine months using the McKenzie exercise program, 60 percent were pain-free, and an additional 27 percent had less pain.) What can you do to speed your recovery from a particular episode or rid yourself of chronic pain?

This chapter is aimed at assisting you to make a more rapid recovery than you have before. In learning how to accelerate your recovery, you will at the same time learn steps you must take in the future if trouble strikes again. And yes, it can happen again. Because once you feel good, you, like all others with the same problem, will tend to forget the precautions you should take. The main thing is to learn how the movements described in this chapter affect your particular back problem.

WHEN YOU ARE IN SIGNIFICANT PAIN

A severe attack of lower back pain may involve pain that is felt at all times regardless of the position you adopt or the movements you perform.

This pain is made much worse by sitting or by arising from a sitting position and bending forward. If the pain is also much worse when you attempt to stand up or walk, and if you are unable to straighten up fully, it may not be possible for you to function, and bed rest is your only alternative.

Recent research tells us that bed rest is not the best option for the treatment of acute and severe back pain and should be used for no more than two days. Those involved in that research, however, may alter their view if they ever personally experience a severe bout of back pain.

In my experience, there are many patients in severe pain who require longer than two days of bed rest before it is possible for them to walk. Nevertheless, early exercise and other movement is preferred for those forced to seek bed rest, and a determined effort to stand upright should be attempted at least once each day.

You may begin the exercise program during your period of bed rest, provided you can lie facedown for short periods. Perform Exercises 1 through 3—Lying Facedown, Lying Facedown in Extension, and Extension in Lying (Figs. 6.1). *These exercises are first-aid for lower back pain.* Immediately following the exercises, roll onto your back and insert the lumbar roll described earlier, under the heading "Correction of Surface." This will maintain your back in the correct position during the period of bed rest.

If your back pain is so severe that it is impossible for you to perform any of the exercises or if your pain is becoming intolerable, seek advice

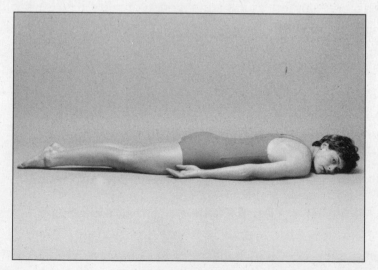

Figure 6.1 *Exercise 1*

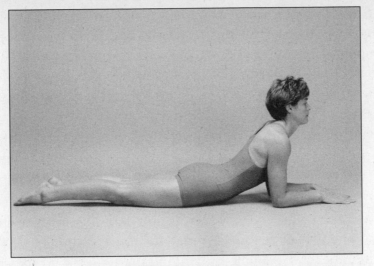

Figure 6.1   *Exercise 2*

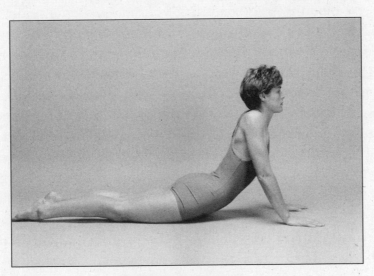

Figure 6.1   *Exercise 3*

from your family physician. Certain over-the-counter (OTC) medications, such as aspirin and other nonsteroidal anti-inflammatory drugs (NSAIDs), one of the best known of which is ibuprofen (found under brand names such as Advil and also available as a less expensive generic drug), may be necessary to provide some relief from pain. Aspirin and other OTC NSAIDs have been found to be highly effective for reducing acute back pain and have fewer side effects than some common prescription drugs. Both aspirin and other NSAIDs have been recommended by the United States federal government's Agency for Health Care Policy and Research.

If your pain is not severe enough to force you to rest in bed, and if you are able to continue with some of your daily activities in spite of your pain, perform Exercises 1 through 3: Lying Facedown, Lying Facedown in Extension, and Extension in Lying.

The aim in performing Exercises 1 through 3 is to restore the lordosis to the fullest possible extent; then we must maintain it by paying careful attention, at all times during the first week, to both posture and movements. Avoid rounded postures that occur when bending or sitting slouched, and in fact sit as little as possible. Therefore, by avoiding flexion, you remove the cause of any further distortion within the joint, and you allow healing to occur. (Remember the example of bending the finger? And the slippery bar of soap?)

When you begin Exercise 3, at first you may experience an increase in pain in the lower back. But as you repeat the exercise, the pain should gradually decrease so that there is significant improvement within a few sessions. The pain may also become more localized in the center of the back (this is the process of centralization, discussed in a previous chapter). This is desirable, as is any movement of pain from the legs and buttocks toward the middle of the back. In time, the pain should disappear and be replaced by a feeling of strain or stiffness, which is more tolerable.

If your pain does not centralize, decrease, or otherwise improve with these exercises, please immediately read "No Response or Benefit," later in this chapter.

As soon as you feel considerably better and no longer have constant pain—perhaps a day or two after you have begun exercising—*you may stop Exercises 1 and 2,* but you must continue Exercise 3 and you must add Exercise 4, Extension in Standing. About this time you must slowly introduce the postural slouch-overcorrect procedure discussed in Chapter 4, because you must now learn to sit correctly and maintain the lordosis just short of its maximum. As a rule, the pain will decrease as the lordosis increases, and you will have no pain at all once you maintain the correct sitting posture. Pain will readily recur if you forget your posture and lose that vital hollow in your lower back. Exercise 4 should be done whenever circumstances keep you from performing Exercise 3: at regular intervals during sitting and working in a stooped position, and before and after lifting as well as during repeated lifting. The slouch-overcorrect procedure must be done two or three times per day until you are familiar with the correct sitting posture.

Once you no longer have acute pain, continue the exercise program as outlined in the next section, When Acute Pain Has Subsided.

WHEN ACUTE PAIN HAS SUBSIDED

For the past few days you have been doing Exercises 1 to 4 and have been maintaining a lordosis at all times. Once the distortion in the joints has decreased and any damaged tissue has healed, you will need to restore your flexibility and recover your normal function. Flexibility is best achieved by doing flexion exercises, which must be performed in such a way that no further damage or tearing occurs within soft tissues that have recently healed. The risks of further damage are much less when the lower back is rounded in the lying position than when it is in the standing position. Therefore you must now do Exercise 5, Flexion in Lying.

You should begin Flexion in Lying when you have mostly recovered from an acute episode of lower back pain and have had long pain-free periods for two to three weeks, even though you may still feel stiffness when you bend forward. Exercise 5 may also be necessary if you have

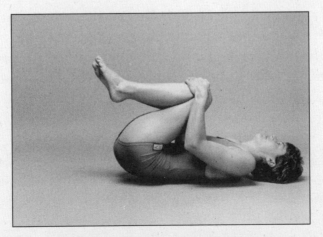

Figure 6.2 *Exercise 5, to be followed by . . .*

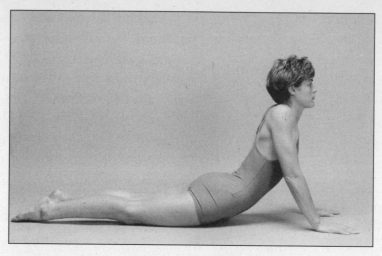

Figure 6.2 ... Exercise 3

improved significantly with Exercises 1 through 4 but after two or three weeks still experience a small amount of pain at the center of your back, pain that seems like it will not disappear.

It is not uncommon for some central, midline, lower back pain to occur when you start Exercise 5, that is, when you do Flexion in Lying. An initial pain that wears off gradually with repetition of the exercise is acceptable; it means that shortened structures are being stretched effectively. *If Exercise 5 causes pain that increases with each repetition, stop.* In this case, it is probably too soon to start flexion and you should wait and try it in another week or two.

When you can touch your chest with your knees easily and without discomfort, you have regained full movement. You may now stop Exercise 5 and begin Exercise 6 (Fig. 6.3). After two to three weeks, Exercise 6 should cause no tightness or discomfort, and once you have reached this point, you may add Exercise 7 to your program (Fig. 6.4).

NOTE: Exercises 5, 6, and 7 should always be followed immediately by Exercise 3, Extension in Lying (Fig. 6.2). In this way, you can rectify any distortion that could develop from Exercises 5, 6, or 7.

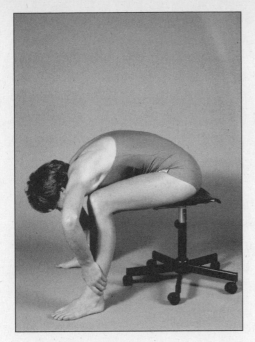

Figure 6.3 *Exercise 6*

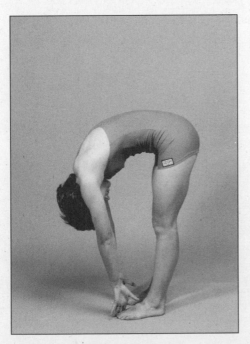

Figure 6.4 *Exercise 7*

Exercise 7 should be carried out at the end of the day once or twice a week to ensure that all the soft tissues in the back remain able to flex. After completing Exercises 5 and 7, follow the guidelines given to prevent recurrence of lower back problems and continue with the exercise program. This is discussed further in the next section, When You Have No Pain or Stiffness.

WHEN YOU HAVE NO PAIN OR STIFFNESS

Many people with lower back problems have long spells in which they experience little or no pain. If, in the past or recently, you have had one or more episodes of lower back pain, start or continue the exercise program even though you may be pain-free at the moment. In this situation it is not necessary to do all the exercises, nor is it necessary to exercise every two hours.

To prevent recurrence of lower back problems:

1. Perform Exercise 3—Extension in Lying—on a regular basis, preferably in the morning and evening.
2. Perform Exercise 4—Extension in Standing—at regular intervals whenever you must sit or bend forward

for long periods. Also do Exercise 4 before and after heavy lifting and during repeated lifting, as well as whenever you feel minor strain developing in your lower back.

3. Practice the slouch-overcorrect procedure (see Chapter 4) whenever you are becoming careless about the correct sitting posture.

4. Perform Exercise 7 once or twice a week to remain fully flexible.

5. Always use a lumbar roll in chairs that do not provide adequate support.

Continue these exercises and adopt them as a regular part of your life. It is essential, however, that you do them *before the onset of pain*. Even more important than exercising, you must watch your posture at all times and never again let postural stresses become the cause of lower back problems. The best exercises will have little or no effect if you constantly fall back into poor posture.

Therefore, you should exercise in the manner described above for the rest of your life, but you *must* develop and maintain good postural habits. Remember, if you lose the lordosis for long periods at a time, you risk the recurrence of lower back pain.

Because it takes only one minute to perform one session of Exercise 3 and two minutes to complete one session of the slouch-overcorrect procedure, lack of time should never be used as an excuse for not being able to do these exercises.

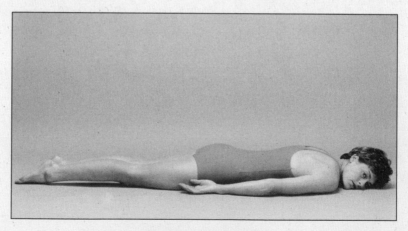

Figure 6.5 Lie face down.

NO RESPONSE OR BENEFIT

After exercising without any relief or benefit for three or four days, you may conclude that the exercises as performed are ineffective. But there are two main causes for lack of response or benefit from the exercises presented in this book.

A lack of response to these exercises is possible in some people whose pain is felt only to one side of the spine, or whose pain is felt much more to one side than the other. If your pain during the course of the day is felt only to one side, or more to one side than the other, or if you feel pain more to one side as you perform Exercises 1, 2, or 3, you may need to modify your body position before you begin these exercises.

Here is how to modify your body position:

1. Position yourself to perform Exercise 1 and allow yourself to relax for a few minutes (Fig. 6.5).
2. Remain facedown, then shift your hips away from the painful side. That is, if your pain usually is more on the right side, you must move your hips three or four inches to the left and once more completely relax for a few minutes (Fig. 6.6).

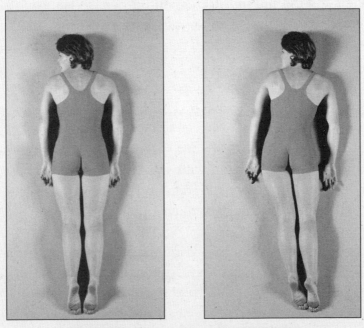

Figure 6.6 Move your hips away from the pain.

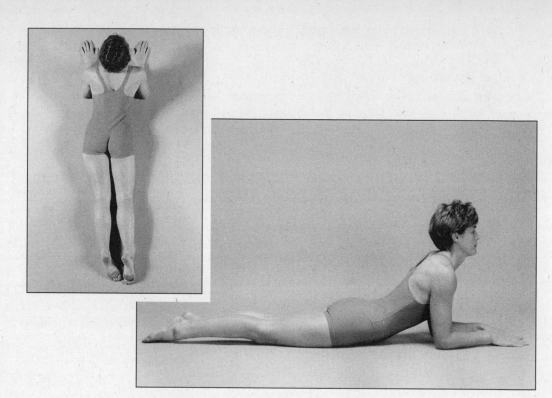

Figure 6.7   *With hips off-center, lean on elbows.*

3.   While allowing the hips to remain off-center, lean on the elbows as described in Exercise 2 and relax for an additional three or four minutes (Fig. 6.7).

You are now ready to begin Exercise 3. With your hips still off-center, complete one session of Exercise 3 (Fig. 6.8) and then relax once more. You may need to repeat the exercise several times, but before beginning each session of 10, ensure that your hips are still off-center: remember, away from the painful side. Even with your hips in the off-center position, try in each repetition to move higher and higher. Reach the maximum amount of extension possible, at which point your arms should be completely straight.

For the next three or four days, continue to perform Exercises 1, 2, and 3 from the modified starting position described in the three steps above. The frequency of the exercises and the number of sessions per day should be the same as recommended in the section titled When You Are in Significant Pain, at the beginning of this chapter.

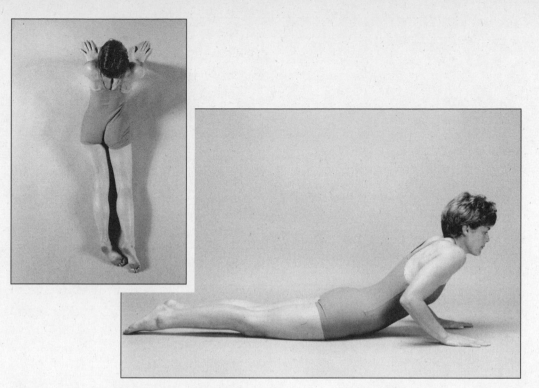

Figure 6.8 *With hips off-center, you are ready to begin Exercise 3.*

After a few days of practice, you may notice that the pain is distributed more evenly across the back or has centralized. Once this occurs, you may stop shifting the hips before exercising and continue exercises as recommended in the section When You Are in Significant Pain. Occasionally, shifting the hips away from the painful side is sufficient to stop the pain completely.

The second cause of lack of response arises when Exercise 3 is done without the pelvis remaining more or less immobilized in a low position. In this case, Exercise 3 occasionally gives benefit for only a few hours, and then the pain returns.

The effectiveness of Exercise 3 can be improved greatly by holding the pelvis down. There are two main ways to do this. Another person can place pressure on your lower back. Or you can construct a simple device for keeping your pelvis in place: you can use an ironing board and either a seat belt or a strong leather belt or strap. Place the belt or strap around the ironing board and your waistline. The added pressure frequently determines whether Exercise 3 succeeds or fails (Fig. 6.9).

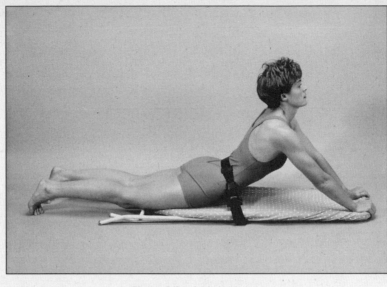

Figure 6.9 Added pressure.

RECURRENCE

Regardless of what you are doing or where you are, at the first sign of recurrence of lower back pain you must take action. That is, you must immediately start the exercises that previously led to recovery, and you must follow the instructions given to relieve acute pain. You must at once begin Exercise 4, Extension in Standing. If this does not eliminate your pain *within minutes*, you must quickly introduce Exercise 3, Extension in Lying. *The immediate use of Exercise 3 very often can prevent the onset of a disabling attack of lower back pain.* If your pain is already too acute to tolerate these exercises, begin with Exercises 1 and 2, Lying Facedown and Lying Facedown in Extension.

Finally, if you have symptoms on one side that do not centralize as a result of the exercises just recommended, shift your hips away from the painful side before beginning the exercises. Further, hold your hips in the off-center position while you exercise. In addition to the exercises, you must pay extra attention to your posture and must maintain the lordosis as much as possible.

If your new episode of lower back pain seems to be different from those you have experienced on other occasions, and if your pain persists despite the fact that you have closely followed the instructions in this book, seek advice from a health professional, ideally a member or associate of the McKenzie Institute.

To obtain the names of credentialed members and associates of the McKenzie Institute, see Appendix A at the back of this book.

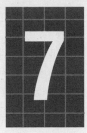

7 Instructions for People with Acute Lower Back Pain

IMMEDIATELY BEGIN THE SELF-TREATMENT EXERCISES

The simple rule is that if bending forward has been the cause of over-stretching, bending backward should rectify this problem and reduce any resultant distortion in the spinal discs. You must restore the lordosis slowly and with caution, never quickly or with jerky movements. You must allow some time for the distorted joint to regain its normal shape and position. A sudden or violent movement may retard this process, increase the strain in and around the affected joint, and thereby result in an increase of lower back pain.

Whenever you are not certain that you recall precisely how to do the exercises, go back to their descriptions in this book and read each line of any exercise you do not recall in detail. Reviewing the exercises is a small price to pay for feeling better. A reminder of Exercises 1, 2, and 3 is found in the photographs at the end of this chapter (Fig. 7.1).

Remember, when you begin the exercises, some increase of midline lower back pain can be expected. Some exercises will be effective only when you actually move into the pain while exercising. You should feel some pain when doing these exercises, but you should never have an increase in pain that lasts into the following day.

When in acute pain, you must, in addition to exercising, make certain adjustments in your daily activities. These adjustments form a very important aspect of self-treatment. If you do not follow the instructions given below, you will unnecessarily delay the healing process. *Following the instructions is entirely your responsibility.*

Maintain your lumbar lordosis at all times. Slouched sitting and bending forward, as when touching the toes, will only increase the pressure in the joints, stretch and weaken the supporting structures, and lead to further damage in the lower back. If you slouch, you will have discomfort and pain. *Good posture is the key to spinal comfort.*

Sit as little as possible, and even then only for short periods. If you must sit, choose a firm, high chair with a straight back, make sure you have an adequate lordosis, and use a lumbar roll to support the lower back. Avoid sitting on a low, soft couch with the legs straight out in front; also avoid sitting up in bed or the bath; all of these situations force you to lose the lordosis.

When getting up from the sitting position, try to maintain the lordosis: move to the front of the seat (or carefully rotate to the exit edge of a seat in a car), stand up by straightening the legs, and avoid bending forward at the waist.

If you have a car, drive it as little as possible. It is better to be a passenger than to be the driver. Whether you are the driver or a passenger, be sure to bring along your lumbar roll. If you must be the driver, your seat should be far enough back from the steering wheel to allow you to drive with your arms relatively straight. With the arms straight, your upper body is held back and you are prevented from slouching; this allows full benefit to be obtained from the lumbar roll.

Avoid activities that require bending forward or stooping. Many activities can be modified enough that you can maintain your lordosis. To the surprise of some, it is possible to maintain the correct standing posture while vacuuming; it is also possible to maintain a correct lordosis when getting down on "all fours" when gardening or making a bed.

If you have acute lower back pain, you should not lift at all. If you must lift, avoid objects that are awkward to handle or are heavier than 30 pounds (about 15 kilograms). At all times you must use the correct lifting technique.

If you are uncomfortable while sleeping or attempting to sleep, you may benefit from a supportive roll around your waist. For most people, the mattress should not be too hard but should be well supported by a firm base. If your bed sags, slats or a sheet of plywood (a "bed board") between

Case History: Hollywood Barbara

Barbara is a Hollywood entertainment executive specializing in the production of documentaries. She works long hours at her desk and also drives to many meetings, screenings, and other events. At age 52, after many years of the same habits, she developed lower back pain that sometimes was sharp. She adapted her chair at work by using a lumbar roll, and after a while rarely had pain at the office.

Her main complaint then became pain while in the car. She didn't have much trouble while driving, but had almost excruciating pain when exiting the vehicle. She was confused about the cause, thinking it must be the exiting rather than the driving.

Her friend Bill sent her the instructions for my exercises. A busy woman who rarely initiates calls, she nevertheless called Bill the day after receiving the exercises. "I'm a lot better!" she exclaimed in relief and surprise. She had been helped by the McKenzie exercises (especially number 3, Extension in Lying). But she also had benefitted from the discussion of the fact that posture is the key to most back pain. She therefore began to use a lumbar roll in the car even though driving rarely was accompanied by pain. The roll helped.

She did best, however, when she paid special attention to the McKenzie Method's advice on how to maintain the lower back lordosis even as one moves from a sitting position to a standing position. In summary, the method says to move to the front of a regular chair or to the exit side of a car seat, then to stand up by straightening the legs, while taking care not to bend forward at the waist. With the combination of lumbar rolls at the office and in the car, the exercises, and the technique for getting out of a sitting posture, Barbara became almost entirely pain-free.

mattress and base will straighten it; as an alternative, you can place the mattress on the floor.

When you have been lying down and you want to get up, keep your back in lordosis: turn on one side, pull both knees up, drop your feet over the edge of the bed, raise yourself to the sitting position by pushing your upper body up with your hands, and avoid bending forward at the waist. Stand up from sitting as described earlier in this chapter.

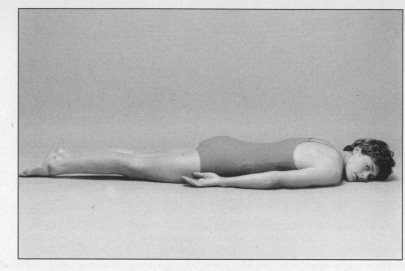

Figure 7.1 *Exercise 1*

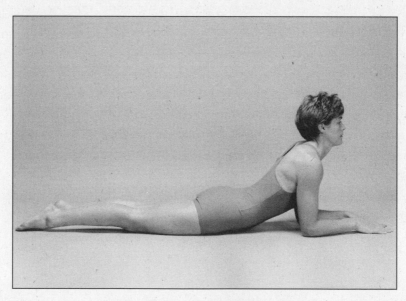

Figure 7.1 *Exercise 2*

Avoid coughing and sneezing while you are sitting or bending forward. If you must cough or sneeze, stand and bend backward.

Avoid those positions and movements that caused your problems in the first place.

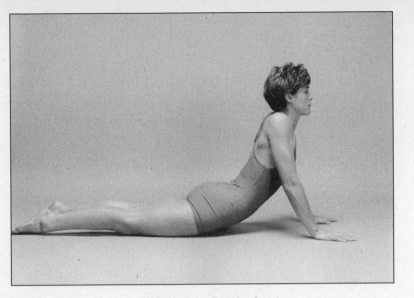

Figure 7.1 Exercise 3

Allow some time for healing to take place.

(In the event you have a sudden onset of acute lower back pain and need a quick, one-page summary of what to do, consult Chapter 15, Panic Page for the Back, which appears on page 185.)

8 Special Back Situations

TREATMENT BY REPEX

Although the system of self-treatment that I have developed is effective for a very high percentage of patients, the success of the method is sometimes limited because of various factors that may prevent the patient from performing the required movements.

Fatigue is probably the limiting factor that patients encounter most commonly. They find they are unable to continue exercising because their arms have become too tired. This is particularly frustrating for the patient whose pain is improving with the exercises but who cannot continue them because of fatigue.

Some patients are unable to relax enough when they perform the push-up exercise (Exercise 3). For the exercise to be effective, it is vital that your lower back be relaxed.

Some patients, especially the elderly, have shoulder, elbow, or wrist problems that keep them from performing the key exercises.

Patients with certain disorders have such restricted movements that the exercises in this book are impossible to perform.

But all is not lost!

To overcome these difficulties, in 1986 I engaged an engineer to develop a machine to provide controlled doses of specific repeated movements for the lower back.

The machine is named REPEX. It can continuously move the lower back many hundreds of times if necessary, without the patient having to exert himself or herself at all. And that's why REPEX has the name it does: it stands for Repeated Endrange Passive EXercise. (Endrange refers to the end of a patient's range of movement.)

The REPEX machine provides a type of treatment known as CPM, or continuous passive motion. Before the development of REPEX, CPM had been found to provide better-quality healing and more rapid recovery when applied to other injured joints of the body. REPEX is the first machine to provide CPM for lower back disorders.

If you have not already resolved your back problem with the McKenzie Method as described in this book, it may well be that the REPEX can assist you further. It is particularly likely that REPEX can help with your problem *if you get relief after each session of exercise but the relief does not last.* In this case, it may well be that an increased number of movements—possible with REPEX—may be all that is required to give you lasting relief.

Treatment by REPEX requires the expertise of a specialist. This treatment is available only through credentialed members and associates of the McKenzie Institute.

To obtain the names of credentialed members and associates of the McKenzie Institute, see Appendix A of this book.

LOWER BACK PAIN IN PREGNANCY

Both during and after pregnancy, women are subjected to altered mechanical stresses that affect the lower back and frequently result in lower back problems. As the new infant develops in the mother's womb, two simple changes occur that influence the woman's posture.

First, there is the gradually increasing bulk and weight of pregnancy. In order to maintain balance during standing and walking, the mother must lean further backward to counterbalance her altered weight distribution. The result of her postural adjustment is an increase in her lordosis. In the final weeks of pregnancy, the lordosis may become excessive, and this may lead to overstretching of the tissues surrounding the joints of the lower back (Fig. 8.0).

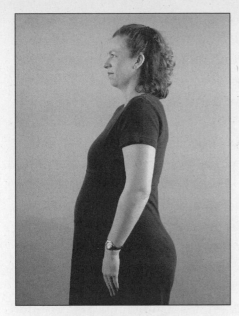

Figure 8.0 *Typical standing position in pregnancy*

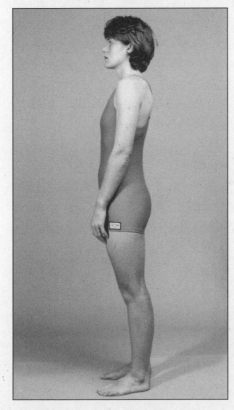

Figure 8.1 *Correct standing posture*

Second, to prepare the body for the impending delivery of the baby, the joints of the pelvis and lower back are made more flexible and elastic through a natural increase in certain hormones. The greater elasticity means that these joints become more lax and are easily overstretched when subjected to mechanical strains.

Once the child is born, the mother is often too busy to care for herself properly, and sometimes the postural fault that has developed during pregnancy remains for the rest of her life.

If your back problems began during or after pregnancy, it is possible that your lordosis has become excessive and that your problems are caused mostly by postural stresses. If this is the case, the extension exercises recommended for most people with lower back pain (Exercises 1–4) are unsuitable for you at the present time. Therefore, if your back problems are caused chiefly by postural factors, you should concentrate mainly on correction of your standing posture (Fig. 8.1). *Problems caused by postural stresses are always resolved by postural correction.*

For one week you must watch your posture very closely. At all times, maintain the correct posture, not only while standing but also while walking. You must *stand tall and walk tall* and not allow yourself to slouch. If, after one week of postural correction, the pain has disappeared or decreased considerably, faulty posture can be blamed for your back problems.

If your back problems began during or after pregnancy and you *feel worse when standing and walking but much better when sitting*, extension exercises are not suitable for you. Now, in addition to the postural correction in standing and walking, perform flexion exercises and self-treatment consisting of Exercises 5 and 6—Flexion in Lying (Fig. 8.2) and Flexion in Sitting (Fig. 8.3).

During the first week, perform Exercise 5 at regular intervals—that is, 10 times per session and six to eight sessions per day. When you have improved to some extent with this procedure, add Exercise 6 in the second week. Exercise 6 must follow Exercise 5 and should be done with the same frequency. *Flexion exercises performed to relieve back pain appearing during pregnancy should not be followed by Extension in Lying.* Once you are completely pain-free, you may stop Exercise 5. In order to prevent recurrence of lower back problems, continue Exercise 6 twice per day, preferably in the morning and evening. At all times, maintain good postural habits, but do *not* use a lumbar roll.

If you are uncertain regarding the category in which you belong— someone who should use flexion exercises or extension exercises—consult a credentialed member or associate of the McKenzie Institute.

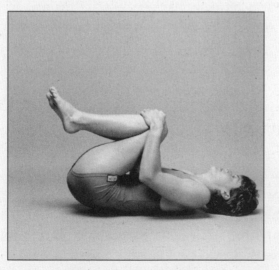

Figure 8.2 Flexion in Lying

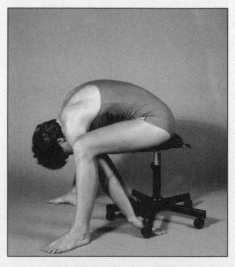

Figure 8.3 Flexion in Sitting

Case History: Adaptations for Pregnancy

Martha is a 33-year-old Georgia policewoman. She began to have lower back pain, radiating into the left thigh, five weeks into a pregnancy, and she knew of no reason for the symptoms. She had the pain while standing and sitting. She saw a doctor 18 weeks into the pregnancy and was told, correctly, that she had a herniated nucleus pulposus.

She tried Exercise 4, Extension in Standing, but it had no effect. Her pregnancy did not permit her to do Exercise 3, Extension in Lying. But a McKenzie-credentialed physical therapist told her she could get most of the benefits of Exercise 3 by adapting it to her pregnancy. He had her stand about two feet from a wall and place her forearms against it. He then had her let her lower back sag as in Exercise 3. After she had done this just 15 times in a single session, her symptoms stopped. Immediately after the exercise, the symptoms were still gone.

The pain would come back from time to time, but doing the adapted Exercise 3 at home helped. A lumbar roll made it possible for her to sit with better posture and less pain.

The same therapist adapted Exercise 5, Flexion in Lying, for use during Martha's pregnancy. Instead of Martha pulling both legs to her chest, the therapist instructed her to pull back one leg at a time. This caused her no pain, and the exercise helped in her recovery.

Throughout the remainder of her pregnancy she was able to keep her symptoms under control, primarily through use of the adapted version of Exercise 3.

LOWER BACK PAIN IN ATHLETES

After 45 years of practice, I have come to the conclusion that lower back problems occurring in athletes—ranging from the professional to the recreational—require more than the usual amount of attention. The symptoms of lower back pain occurring in athletes can often behave in a fashion that is extremely mystifying and confusing. A combination of several factors adds to the confusion.

First, athletes are highly motivated to participate in their treatment and sometimes, in an attempt to speed their recovery, carry to excess the advice given to them. Their overexuberant participation in the rehabilitation of their back problems very often *delays rather than accelerates* the healing process.

A second important point is that the athlete's enthusiasm to participate in his or her favorite pastime or sport often leads him or her to return to full participation long before there has been sufficient time for complete healing.

A third and certainly the most common source of confusion can stem from the widespread belief among athletes that the sole cause of their problem lies in their frequent participation in a particular sporting activity. Later, this belief is reinforced by a health professional, who all too often comes to the same conclusion. It is not difficult to reach this conclusion, for probably three out of five athletes who experience lower back pain state that their pain appears after they have participated in a sport or have engaged in some equally vigorous activity.

All this comes from a mistaken effort at logic that plagues people who try to analyze their health care problems. The Latin for it is *post hoc, ergo propter hoc,* meaning "after this, therefore because of this." *Merriam Webster's Collegiate Dictionary* defines the phrase as "relating to or being the fallacy of arguing from temporal sequence to a causal relation."

If your back began hurting an hour after your friend called you on the phone, would you say that the call with the friend injured your back? This is an extreme and silly example of the logical fallacy just described. But the fact is that people, including not just back sufferers but also their health care professionals, tend to believe that when back pain follows an activity that involves the back—even if it involves the back in good posture—the pain is due to the activity.

Many athletic careers have stopped for weeks or months or permanently because of *post hoc, ergo propter hoc.* Let's be sure that you don't stop your activity because of a logical fallacy. The belief that pain appearing shortly after activity must be caused by the activity itself is widespread and understandable but unfortunately is frequently mistaken.

Often, the true cause of pain in athletes is that they adopt a slouched position after they have, in their athletic endeavor, thoroughly exercised their joints (Fig. 8.4). After exertion, we usually sit down and relax: because we are tired, we almost immediately adopt the relaxed sitting posture. In other words, after vigorously exercising, we collapse "in a heap" and slouch badly.

During vigorous exercise the joints of the spine are moved rapidly in many directions over an extended period of time. This process causes a thorough stretching in all directions of the soft tissues surrounding the joints. In addition, the fluid gel contained in the spinal discs is loosened, and it seems that distortion or displacement can occur if, after exercise, an exercised joint is placed in an extreme posture. This is very often the cause of back pain in athletes, and the cause-and-effect relationship can be proven rather easily, as will be explained.

If lower back pain has in fact occurred as a result of participation in a sport, it would be appropriate to recommend rest from the activity. But if the pain has appeared *after the activity has been completed and as a result of adopting a slouched sitting posture, resting would be entirely inappropriate.* To advise an athlete to cease participation in his or her favorite pastime can have serious consequences, both emotional and physical.

If you are an athlete, or if you participate in vigorous non-athletic activities, and you have recently developed lower back pain, it is necessary to discover the true cause of your problem. In order to treat your condition

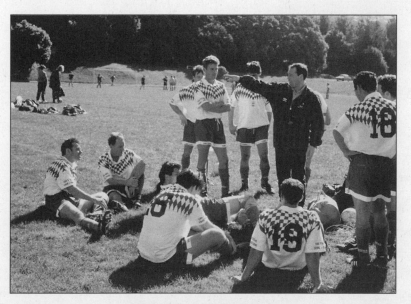

Figure 8.4 *Slouched positions*

correctly and successfully, *we must determine whether your pain appeared during the particular activity or afterward.*

If the pain appeared *during* the activity itself, your sport may well be the cause of the present problems. You may remember something that happened at the time of the activity and can describe what you felt at that moment. But a very large percentage of people who have back pain and participate in a sport never feel discomfort or pain while they are participating; their pain appears *after* the activity.

It's easy to determine if your lower back problems are the result of slouched sitting that has occurred after athletic or other activity. From now on, *immediately after the activity,* watch your posture closely and sit correctly with the lower back in moderate lordosis and supported by a lumbar roll (Fig. 8.5).

For example, if you have finished a few sets of tennis, a game of football, or a round of golf, do not then sink into a comfortable lounge chair, or slouch on a nearby patch of grass, or slouch in the car as you drive home. Instead, sit correctly, with your posture maintained precisely (Fig. 8.6).

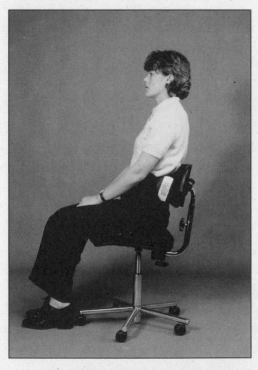

Figure 8.5 *Lower back in moderate lordosis, supported by lumbar roll*

If, with this extra postural care, no pain occurs after a sports activity that previously was followed by back problems, the answer to your problem is clear and the responsibility for preventing further trouble is entirely your own.

If you fall into the group of people who develop pain only after activity, do not begin the McKenzie Method exercises at the same time that you begin correcting your posture. If the exercises are performed in conjunction with postural correction, it is impossible to determine whether you improved because of the postural correction or the exercises.

If your pain continues to appear after activity in spite of correcting your posture, it is possible that at some point during or before the activity you weakened or damaged some of the soft tissues in your lower back. If this is the case, *now* is the time to begin self-treatment. To do this, perform Exercises 3 and 4—Extension in Lying and Extension in Standing—on a regular basis.

Poor posture is often seen in athletes during intervals of non-participation: for example, when waiting their turn to come to the plate in baseball or to practice free throws in basketball. It is necessary to maintain good posture during these intervals as well as after completion of the activity.

If your pain appears regularly *while* you run or jog, you should begin the self-treatment program outlined in Chapter 7, Instructions for People with Acute Lower Back Pain. You should also seek advice about the type of shoes you wear, the surfaces you run on, and, possibly, your running technique. If your problems persist despite following the advice in Chapter 7, you may need special treatment.

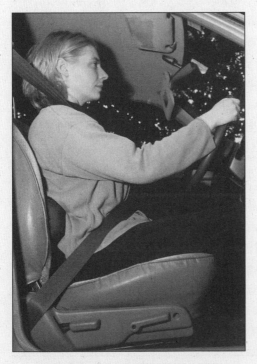

Figure 8.6 *Driving with correct posture*

LOWER BACK PAIN IN THE ELDERLY

It is now known that acute lower back pain tends to occur less frequently in each person once we pass the age of 55. So if you are over 55 (or even a little younger), you may notice that you experience a more persistent ache in the lower back than you previously had but that you no longer have the acute and severe episodes that affected you when you were younger. Nevertheless, this aching can cause significant problems, especially if you are forced to reduce activity. The human body thrives on activity and decays with prolonged inactivity. It is undesirable for any of us, regardless of age, to reduce our levels of activity. Only if

Case History: Journal

Herb, a New York journalist, was also a long-distance runner. From ages 28 to 34, he completed seven marathons; his only pain was from sore legs and a chafed toe. But during a vacation when he was 44, he ran one rigorous but short (1.7-mile) race in California's Sierra Nevada. He was pain-free during the event, but was so exhausted by running hard at high altitude that, right after the race, he bent over for about two minutes, his hands on his knees. While doing this, he suddenly had severe pain in the middle of the lower back, pain that did not go away even when he resumed a normal standing posture.

Herb could not walk a step without sharp pain and needed a ride back to the start of the race (he had planned to walk). He naturally assumed that running had caused the pain, and he was afraid he would have to give up this form of exercise. A cousin told Herb about the McKenzie exercises and that the McKenzie Method says that when one has no pain while exercising but has pain directly thereafter, the culprit is almost always poor posture after exercise rather than the exercise itself: the exercise merely makes the athlete more vulnerable to the problems that can be caused by poor posture.

After his first set of McKenzie exercises, Herb's pain became much better; he was helped especially by Exercise 3, Extension in Lying, and Exercise 5, Flexion in Lying. He also learned the importance of maintaining good posture in standing or sitting after hard exercise. He soon was able to return to running. With attention to post-running posture, Herb never again had back pain following training runs or races.

reduced activity is forced upon us by significant health-related problems should we exercise less.

A health professional may tell you that you have "degenerative" changes in your back or that you have arthritis and will "just have to live with it." *While it may be true that your back has worn somewhat with aging, it certainly is not true that you will "just have to live with it."* It has been found that many people who have spinal joints that are worn with age have never had back pain, and we now know that the wear is not, by itself, a cause of pain.

In my experience, there are few people who would not derive some benefit from this book's advice about posture or the exercises, or both. Every older person should carry out the advice on the correction of the sitting, standing, and lying postures.

Not all of you in the older group will be able to perform each exercise as advised, but all of you should *try*. I have found that age is not necessarily a barrier to the successful application of the exercises. Although there are some who may not succeed because of weakness or disability, most will be able to advance at least partway through the recommended program.

My advice to you is to consider starting the exercise program by reducing the number of exercises to be done in each session and to do fewer sessions in the course of a day. Don't hurry the process, and always rest adequately after completing the exercises—properly supported in the correct position, of course!

OSTEOPOROSIS

From middle age on, many women are affected by a disorder called osteoporosis. This is essentially a mineral-deficiency disorder. During and after menopause there is a significant and continuing deficiency in calcium replacement. As a result, many women must take calcium tablets on a regular basis. Because of calcium deficiency, there is a weakening of bone structure that results in a slow but progressive reduction in bone density. This in turn allows the postures of those with osteoporosis to become extremely rounded, especially in the middle—*thoracic*—part of the spine.

In persons affected by this disorder, there are risks of fractures occurring without significant forces being applied to the vertebrae. Research conducted at the Mayo Clinic in the United States found that extension exercises performed regularly (Fig. 8.7) significantly reduced the number of compression fractures in the group performing such exercises. A similar group exercising differently and a group not exercising at all had significantly more fractures when examined at least one year after the beginning of the study. The Mayo study suggests that women from about the age of 40 onward should practice extension exercises on a regular basis.

Here is how to do the exercise found so effective in the Mayo study:

Lie facedown with a pillow under your abdomen. With the hands clasped behind the neck or behind the lower back, lift the top half of your body. At the same time, lift both legs, remembering to keep them straight. After lifting the body and legs as high as possible, gradually lower both and relax for one second.

The exercise should be repeated until the back muscles feel fatigued and the exercise is becoming difficult to continue. The exercise should be performed 15 to 20 times, four or five times per week, for about a month. After that time you should gradually increase the number of exercises until you are doing 50 to 60 at a time. You should do the Mayo exercise for the rest of your life!

If you are uncertain regarding how to follow this advice, discuss it with your doctor before beginning the program. If you have difficulties with the exercises for one reason or another, consult a McKenzie-credentialed physical therapist or chiropractor who can show you ways to modify the exercises without necessarily reducing their effectiveness.

The muscles you strengthen by doing the exercise recommended by the Mayo Clinic study are also the muscles responsible for holding you upright. Maintaining good posture at all times will probably assist in the strengthening process. Good posture may also reduce the likelihood of small fractures.

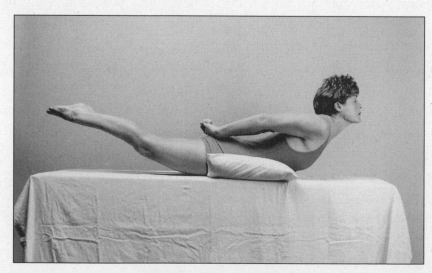

Figure 8.7   *Mayo Clinic exercise*

Common Back Remedies and Solutions

MEDICINES AND DRUGS

As mentioned earlier in this book, most of the common back pains we experience are mechanical in origin and therefore are affected only by those drugs and medications that are able to relieve pain. There are no medicines or drugs able to remove the *causes* of our common backaches and pains. Therefore, medication should be taken only when your pains are severe or when you must find relief.

Certain medications such as aspirin and other nonsteroidal anti-inflammatory drugs (NSAIDs) have been found to be the most useful for alleviating acute back pain and have fewer side effects than some commonly prescribed medications. Both have been recommended by the United States federal government's Agency for Health Care Policy and Research.

BED REST

When your back pain is so severe that bed rest is required, you should restrict this period of rest, if at all possible, to two or three days.

A recent study conducted in the United States demonstrated that those patients resting in bed for two days recovered as well as those who stayed in bed for seven days. But patients who continued to walk and move were able to go back to work sooner than those who rested for either two or seven days. (Deyo, R. A. et al.: "How Many Days of Bed Rest for Acute Low Back Pain?" *New England Journal of Medicine,* 1986, 315: 1064–1070.) And I have seen many patients who could still not get out of bed after 10 days.

ACUPUNCTURE

Acupuncture can relieve pain and, when all else has failed, is well worth a trial. You should be aware, however, that as with taking medications, acupuncture can give you relief, but it cannot correct the underlying mechanical problem.

CHIROPRACTIC

In the past the treatment of back and neck problems by the adjustment or manipulation of the spine was one of the most popular forms of treatment. In addition, it was demonstrated by chiropractors and osteopaths in the first half of the twentieth century that a short-term benefit could be obtained through this form of treatment. Nevertheless, much research has now shown that spinal manipulation and adjustment provide no long-term benefit. Also, the use of either technique can create a dependency.

A recent study by internationally renowned researchers at the University of Washington has shown that one month after completing treatment, patients who had been taught the McKenzie Method improved to the same degree as did patients receiving manipulation by chiropractors. *But the patients using the McKenzie Method underwent fewer treatments to achieve the same improvement. Also, 72 percent of the McKenzie patients reported that in the event of recurrence of their back pain, they would be able to manage their own problems.* This has great significance for patients with recurring problems.

About 80 percent of patients with common back problems can benefit from being taught the self-manipulation and postural methods outlined in this book. The other 20 percent of the population are the only ones who may require any form of manipulative therapy.

It is important that people who are suffering from back pain understand that spinal manipulation or adjustments should not be given to the whole population with back pain for the purpose of ensuring that it is delivered to the relative few who really need it. This would be like giving surfboards to every citizen of every one of the 50 states so that it was certain that those who might use them—a relative few living mostly on the coasts of California and Hawaii—would receive them. Spinal manipulation certainly should not be used unless self-treatment measures have already been tried and been found to be unsuccessful.

Manipulative physical therapists, chiropractors, and osteopaths all dispense spinal manipulation or adjustment. The techniques used by the three groups are similar. Nevertheless, the theory and rationale for providing these procedures differ completely among the three groups.

Manipulative physical therapists and chiropractors who are members or associates of the McKenzie Institute are well versed in the entire range of mechanical treatments that are in use for back pain today. (See Appendix A.)

Not all chiropractors use the procedures in this book, but several chiropractic colleges in the United States are now teaching the methods through faculty members of the McKenzie Institute.

ELECTROTHERAPY

In 1995, the United States federal government's Agency for Health Care Policy and Research published a list of recommendations to guide health professionals involved in acute back care. Because there was no supportive scientific evidence, the agency could not recommend various forms of heat, shortwave and microwave diathermy, and ultrasound, all of which are commonly used in the treatment of back pain.

You should be aware that these treatments provide no long-term benefit and do nothing to treat the underlying problem; nor is there any scientific evidence that they accelerate healing.

BACK PAIN IN THE COMMUNITY

Lower back pain is widespread throughout the world, both in Western and Eastern cultures. In Western countries, in which more data are available, approximately 80 percent of people will at least one time in their lives suffer a back pain episode so severe as to require bed rest.

Many things could be done to improve this situation. You as an individual should complain whenever you find inappropriate seating in public offices or buildings or in public transit vehicles. If your car's seats are inadequate, you should complain to your car dealer; better still, look for another car or consider having your car retrofitted with better seats.

I was about to write, "When choosing lounge furniture...," but an American friend of mine has advised me that in the U.S. a "lounge" generally is a bar or a women's rest room. So I will re-phrase. I mean to comment on furniture used for relaxing at home. So I will say that when choosing *living room* furniture (which nearly always seems designed to cause or perpetuate back problems), you should persist until you find chairs that are properly designed. When you are in a furniture store and find seating that is poorly designed, you should tell management there that this is the case. If you complain either to a car dealer or a furniture store manager, nothing will change instantly. But enough complaints can result in reform.

Few airlines provide seating that adequately supports the lower back. This has serious consequences for some individuals who must fly long distances over a period of many hours.

Office workers should demand seating that provides adequate lumbar support. There are many sophisticated-looking and expensive office and secretarial chairs on the market that provide no lumbar support whatsoever. On the other hand, chairs that provide good support can often be found at moderate prices.

Although poor seating design is a major factor contributing to the development of lower back pain, another, more important factor is becoming increasingly evident. Where once our school physical education instructors were concerned with poor posture in our children and corrected it when they saw it, they now seem more interested in producing the best football team, the highest-scoring basketball player, and the fastest sprinter. Physical education teachers in all parts of the world no longer seem to equip our children with the information that is so necessary if they are to care for their own physical needs during a lifetime on this planet.

Spinal pain of postural origin would not occur if this basic education were given to individuals at an early age. Ask any 12-year-old child if he or she has been shown at school how to stand correctly or how to sit correctly. Chances are that the child will tell you that he or she has never been shown either of these two fundamental postures. Similarly, chances are slim that the child has been told about the harmful consequences that may occur if posture is neglected.

If these matters are of concern to you, you might politely request that your school administration or P.E. teachers make postural physical education a priority. In addition, you might suggest that administrators evaluate school furniture for its effects on posture. Good postural habits must be instilled at an early age.

These are steps that you as a concerned individual can take to help to bring about some of the changes that must occur if society is to grapple sensibly with the enormous problem of back pain. In the United States alone, this problem costs from $50 to $70 billion a year in everything from medical expenses to days lost from work.

For information on the McKenzie Institute Postural Video, which is available to schools, please see Appendix A.

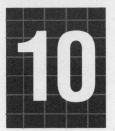 **Neck Problems**

Neck problems come with many names. Arthritis in the neck. Spondylosis of the neck. Rheumatism. Fibrositis. Slipped disc. And, when they involve pain extending into the arm, neuritis and neuralgia.

At some time during our lives, most of us suffer from pain in the neck or from pain originating in the neck that is felt across the shoulders, in a shoulder blade, or in the upper or lower arm. Pain coming from the neck can also be felt as far away as the hand, and symptoms such as "pins and needles" and numbness can be felt in the fingers. Some people suffer from headaches that can be traced to problems in the neck.

Usually the aches and pains occur intermittently. That is, there are times in the day when no pain is felt, or there are whole days when no pain is felt. The symptoms may appear mysteriously, often for no apparent reason. And just as enigmatically the symptoms may vanish.

These aches and pains also may occur constantly. That is, for some patients pain is felt at all times, to one degree or another. People who have pain all the time frequently are forced to take pills. Nevertheless, it is uncommon for these people to have to stop work, though even this occasionally does occur. More often, the pain simply makes their lives miserable and they must reduce their activities in order to keep their discomfort at a moderate level. Therefore neck problems can seriously affect their lifestyle.

If you have neck problems, you may already have discovered that symptoms can in some cases last for months or even years. Or you may have found that treatments often are able to stop your pain, but that the pain returns later. You may be reading this book because you have persistent pains that have not disappeared, despite the fact that you have received the best of treatment.

Whatever the situation, you most likely will realize that many of the treatments dispensed by doctors, physical therapists, and chiropractors are prescribed for your present symptoms and are not directed at preventing future problems. Time and again you may have to seek assistance to get relief from your neck pain.

How good it would be if you were able to treat yourself whenever pain were to return! Better yet, how good it would be if you could apply a system of treatment to yourself that would prevent pain from coming back!

But I am not writing about some dream world that does not exist; I am not describing some old black-and-white episode of *The Twilight Zone*. In fact, beginning around the early 1970s, methods have been discovered that enable us to manage our own spinal problems. Unfortunately, however, this information has been much like a well-kept secret. It was not widely disseminated among health professionals until the 1980s. This is because, like many developments in medicine, new ideas must be shown to be effective before they are widely adopted.

The method I have developed has been used by doctors and physical therapists in many parts of the world since the early 1970s, and generally their patients are achieving the same happy results.

One of the main points of this book is that, just as with the back, the management of the neck is *your* responsibility. If, for some reason or other, *you* have developed neck problems, then *you* must learn how to deal with your present symptoms and how to prevent future problems. Self-treatment will be more effective in the long-term management of your neck pain than any other form of therapy.

Despite its value to most neck patients, this book is not meant for you, at least not at this stage, if you have developed neck pain for the first time and it is no better 10 days after onset. In that case, consult your doctor, who will evaluate your neck problems from various medical angles. When appropriate, he or she will refer you to a physical therapist (ideally a McKenzie-credentialed one) for treatment and, more important, for advice and instructions on how to prevent further neck problems. You should also seek advice from your doctor if there are complications to your neck problems. Examples of complications are severe, stabbing pains, or that your head is pulled off-center, or that you have severe, continuing headaches.

Finally, this book will help 80 percent of people with neck pain, which is to say that it will not help 20 percent. This book is meant for those with straightforward mechanical problems, which are by far the most common cause of neck pain. I hope you fall into this category and that you will therefore benefit greatly from this book.

THE CERVICAL SPINE

The technical name for the series of vertebrae in the neck is the *cervical spine*. As you will recall from Chapter 2, the spine (Fig. 10.1) consists of 33 bones called vertebrae. The top seven are the cervical vertebrae. These rest upon one another like a stack of spools. Each vertebra has a solid part in front, called the vertebral body, and a hole in the back (Fig. 10.2). When lined up as the spinal column, these holes form the spinal canal. This canal serves as a protected passageway for the spinal cord, the bundle of nerves that extends from head to pelvis.

Separating the vertebrae are special cartilages called the discs. These are located between the vertebral bodies, just in front of the spinal cord. (Fig. 10.2). Each disc consists of a soft fluid center part, the *nucleus*. The nucleus is surrounded and held together by a cartilage ring, called the *annulus* or *annular ligament*. The discs are like rubber washers and act as shock absorbers. They are able to alter their shape, thus allowing movement of one vertebra on another and allowing movement of the neck as a whole.

The vertebrae and the discs are linked by a series of joints to form the cervical spine. Each joint is held together by its surrounding soft tissues, that is, by a capsule reinforced by *ligaments*. Muscles lie over one or more joints of the neck and may extend upward to the head or downward to the trunk. At each end, each muscle changes into a tendon by which it attaches itself to different bones. When a muscle contracts, it causes movement in one or more joints.

Between each two vertebrae are two small openings, one on either side. Through these openings, the left and right spinal nerves leave the spinal canal (Fig. 10.3). Among other tasks, the spinal nerves supply our

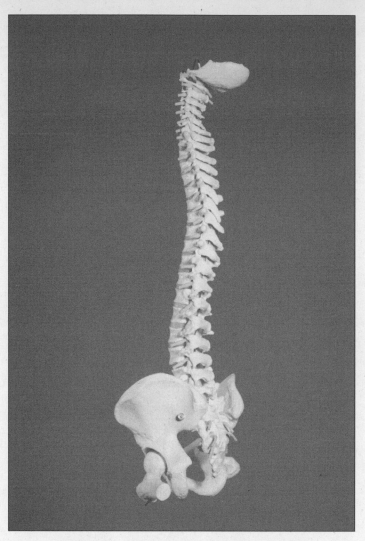

Figure 10.1 *The human spine viewed from the side.*

muscles with power and our skin with sensation. The nerves are really part of our alarm system: pain is the warning that a structure is about to be damaged or has already sustained some damage.

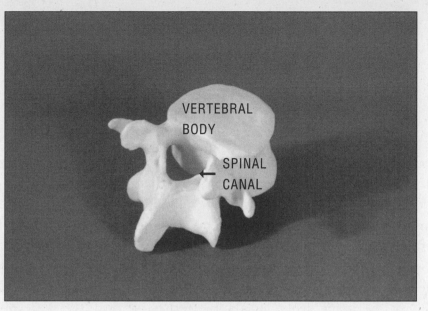

Figure 10.2   A vertebra

FUNCTIONS OF THE CERVICAL SPINE

On top of this complex of bones and "washers" rests the head. The head contains our computer system, better known as the brain, as well as important sensors associated with it such as the eyes, ears, nose, and mouth. The vertebrae, the discs, and the head form a series of flexible joints that allow the head to turn almost 180 degrees from one side to the other, to look up and down, and to tilt left and right. In addition, the head can adopt many positions that are combinations of the movements mentioned above.

The main functions of the cervical spine are:

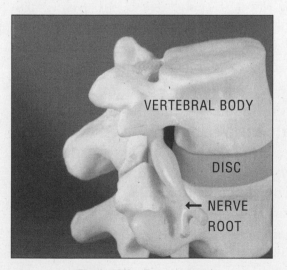

Figure 10.3   Two vertebrae

• To support the head

- To allow it to move in many directions and adjust its position in fine degrees in order to assist the working of the sensors

- To provide a protected passageway for the bundle of nerves that extends from the brain to the sacrum, which is the tail end of the spine

The neck has a high degree of flexibility due to the "specially designed" structure of the joints, in particular those between the uppermost vertebrae and the head. Its flexibility is further increased because in this area no bony structures are attached to the spine. Therefore the neck can move relatively more freely than the rest of the spine, whose movements are restricted by the rib cage and the pelvis. On the other hand, because the neck is not surrounded and supported by these structures, it is also more vulnerable than the rest of the spine when it is subjected to strains. The very flexibility of the neck, so helpful and so necessary for everyday living, is also the cause of many of our problems. The wide range of movement of the neck exposes it to an equally wide range of stresses and strains.

NATURAL POSTURE

A side view of the human body (Fig. 10.4) shows that there is a small inward curve in the neck just above the shoulder girdle. Can you guess what this inward curve is called? It's a word you certainly have heard enough in this book. Yes, it's called a lordosis. When we discussed the back, we repeatedly referred to the *lumbar* lordosis. The inward curve in your neck is called the *cervical* lordosis. This curve in the cervical spine is our main concern in this "neck part" of this book.

The shoulder girdle consists of the left and right *scapulas* (shoulder blades) and the left and right *clavicles* (collar bones). When you stand upright, your head should be directly above the shoulder girdle, therefore forming a small but visible lordosis (Fig. 10.4). Due to postural neglect, people can often be seen with their heads in front of their bodies, with their chins poking forward. (Fig. 10.5). When this is the case, the cervical lordosis is altered in shape and the joints are distorted. In this position, the joints of the lower neck are bent relatively forward (flexed), whereas the joints between the upper part of the neck and the head are bent backward (extended). This is called the "protruded head posture" (Fig. 10.5) and, if present often enough and long enough, can cause neck pain to develop.

WHY NECK PAIN?

Mechanical pain occurs when the joint between two bones has been placed in a position that overstretches the surrounding soft tissues. This is true for mechanical pain in any joint of the body, but in the spine there are additional factors. Here the tissues that surround the joints between the vertebrae, in particular the tissues in the ligaments, are also responsible for supporting the soft discs that separate the vertebrae. These tissues hold the discs in an enclosed compartment and help to form a shock-absorbing mechanism.

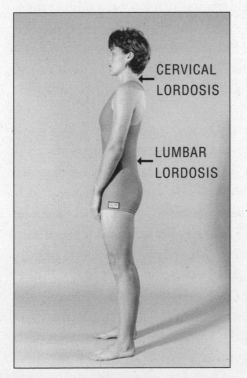

CERVICAL
LORDOSIS

LUMBAR
LORDOSIS

Figure 10.4
Good posture, featuring the cervical lordosis

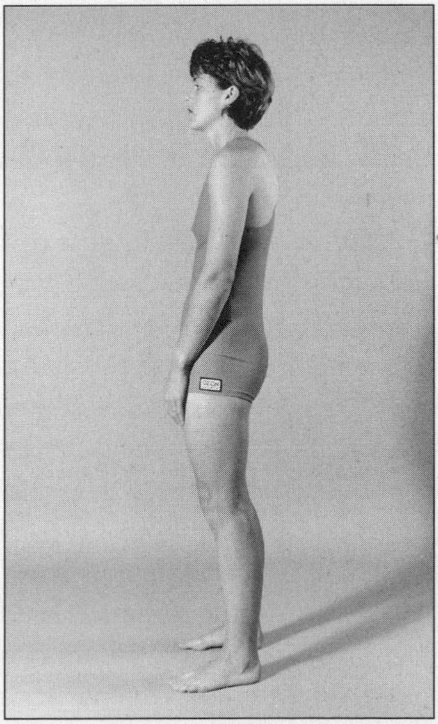

Figure 10.5
Bad posture, with the head protruding

Pain of mechanical origin may arise in the neck for the following reasons:

- The ligaments and other soft tissues that hold the vertebrae together can simply be overstretched without further damage.

- Overstretching may be caused by an outside force placing a sudden, severe strain on the neck. Examples are injuries caused by auto accidents and contact sports. This type of stress cannot always be avoided, as it occurs unexpectedly and takes a person unawares.

- Most often, overstretching is caused by postural stresses that place less severe strains on the neck over a longer period of time. This type of stress is one that *we exert on our own neck*, and therefore we can easily influence it. Here lies our main responsibility in the self-treatment and prevention of neck pain.

Complications arise when overstretching of soft tissues leads to actual tissue damage. It is often thought that neck pain is caused by strained muscles. Muscles, which are the source of power and cause movement, can indeed be overstretched and thereby injured. But muscle injury requires a considerable amount of external force and does not happen all that often. In addition, muscles usually heal rapidly and seldom cause pain lasting for more than a week or two.

On the other hand, whenever the impact of the injuring force is severe enough to affect the muscles, the underlying soft tissues such as the capsule and ligaments will be damaged as well. In fact, usually these two are damaged long before the muscles are. When these tissues heal, they may form scar tissues, become less elastic, and shorten. At this stage even normal movements may stretch the scars in these shortened structures and produce pain. Unless appropriate exercises are performed to gradually stretch and lengthen these structures and restore their normal flexibility, they may become a continuous source of neck pain or headache.

Complications of another nature arise when the ligaments surrounding the disc are injured to such an extent that the disc loses its ability to absorb shock and its outer wall is weakened. This allows the soft inside of the disc to bulge outward and, in extreme cases, to burst through the outer ligament, which may cause serious problems. When the disc bulge protrudes far enough backward, it may press painfully on the spinal nerve. This may cause some of the pains felt well away from the source of the trouble, for example in the arm or hand.

Due to this bulging, the disc may become severely distorted and prevent the vertebrae from lining up properly during movement. In this case, some movements may be blocked partially or completely, and forcing these movements causes severe pain. This is the reason that some people can hold the head only in an off-center position. Those of you who experience a sudden onset of pain and following this are unable to move the head in a normal way may have some bulging of the soft disc material. This need not be cause for alarm. The movements described in this book, and especially the seven exercises for the neck, are carefully designed to reduce any disturbance of this nature.

POSTURAL STRESSES

The most common form of neck pain is caused by the overstretching of ligaments due to postural stresses. This may occur when you sit with poor

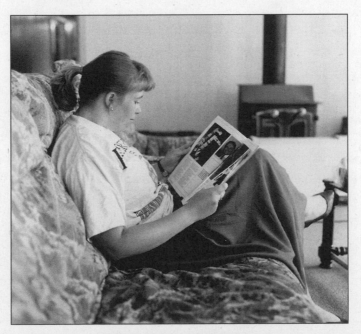

Figure 10.6 *Bad sitting posture*

posture for a long time (Fig. 10.6); when you lie or sleep through the night with your head in an awkward position (Figs. 10.7 and 10.7a), and when you work in strained positions (Fig. 10.8).

Of all these postural stresses, the one that is by far most often at fault is poor sitting posture, that is, sitting with the head protruded. Poor posture may produce neck pain all by itself. But once neck problems have developed, poor posture will frequently make them worse and will always make them last longer than they otherwise would have.

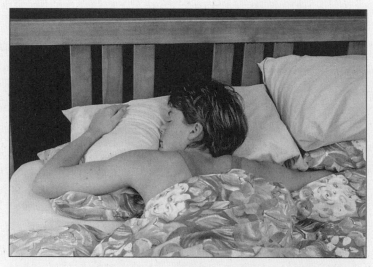

Figure 10.7   *Bad sleeping position*

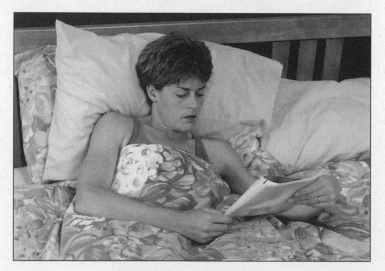

Figure 10.7a   *Bad lying position*

The main theme of this chapter is that if you avoid prolonged over-stretching, pain of postural origin will not occur. If pain does develop, there are certain movements—and in particular certain exercises—you can perform in order to stop the pain. You should not have to seek assistance whenever postural pain arises.

WHERE THE PAIN IS FELT

The sites of pain caused by neck problems vary from one person to another. In a first attack, pain is usually felt at or near the base of the neck, in the center (Fig. 10.9) or just to one side (Fig. 10.10). Usually the pain subsides within a few days. In subsequent attacks, pain may reach across both shoulders (Fig. 10.11), to the top of one shoulder, or to the shoulder blade (Fig. 10.12). Later still, pain may reach the outside or back of the upper arms as far as the elbow (Fig. 10.13), or it may extend below the elbow to the wrist or hand, and you may feel "pins and needles," or numbness, in the fingers (Fig. 10.14). As a result of neck problems, some people experience headaches. Often these headaches are felt at the top of the neck and at the base and back of the head, on one or both sides (Fig. 10.15). But they also can spread from the back of the head over the top of the head to above or behind the eye, again on one or both sides (Fig. 10.16).

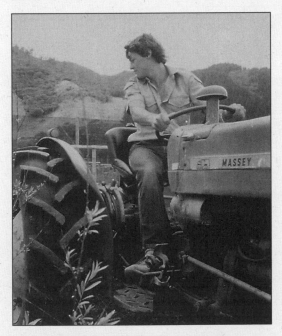

Figure 10.8   *Strained working position*

WHO CAN PERFORM SELF-TREATMENT?

Only relatively few people with neck pain will not benefit from the advice given in this book. Nearly everyone can begin the exercise

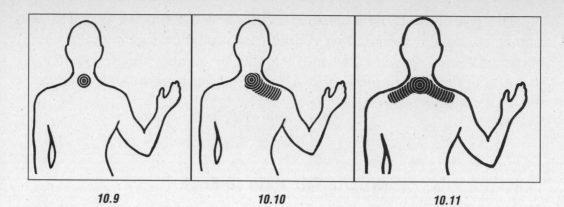

10.9   10.10   10.11

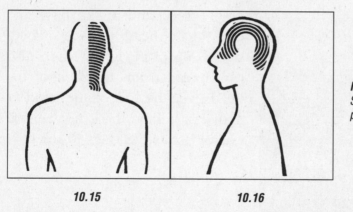

10.12   10.13   10.14

10.15   10.16

Figure 10.9–10.16
Sites of pain caused by neck problems

program, provided the recommended precautions are taken. Once you have started the exercises, carefully watch your pain pattern. If your pains are getting progressively worse, and remain worse the following day, you should stop the exercises and get advice from your doctor or McKenzie-credentialed physical therapist.

In any of the following situations, you should not begin the exercise program without first consulting your doctor or physical therapist:

- If you have developed neck pain for the first time and it is no better 10 days after onset

- If you have pain near or at the wrist or hand and experience sensations of "pins and needles," or numbness, in the fingers

- If you have developed neck problems following a recent, severe accident

- If you recently have developed headaches. In this case, your eyes or eyeglasses may need to be checked.

- If you experience severe headaches that have come on for no apparent reason, have never gone away, and are gradually getting worse

- If you have episodes of severe headaches that are accompanied by nausea and dizziness

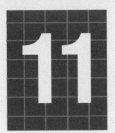

Common Causes of Neck Pain

1. SITTING FOR PROLONGED PERIODS

When we are moving about, especially when we walk briskly, we assume a fairly upright posture. Our head is retracted and held directly over the vertebral column and consequently receives the maximum possible support. When we sit and relax in a chair (Fig. 11.1), the head and neck slowly protrude, because the muscles that support them get tired. As the muscles tire, they relax, and we lose the main support for good posture.

The result is the protruded head posture (Fig. 11.1a). This posture can be seen around us every day. It is not present during infancy, but develops from the mid-teen years onward. We are not really designed to sit for six to eight hours daily, five to six days a week.

When the protruded head posture is maintained long enough, it causes overstretching of the ligaments. As a result, pain will arise *only in certain positions.* Once the protruded posture has become a habit and is maintained most of the time, it may also cause distortion of the discs in the vertebral joints. At this stage, *movements as well as positions* will produce pain. Neck problems developed this way are the result of postural neglect. Poor neck posture is not the only cause of neck pain. It is, however, one of the main causes and is the most troublesome factor in causing neck pain to go on and on.

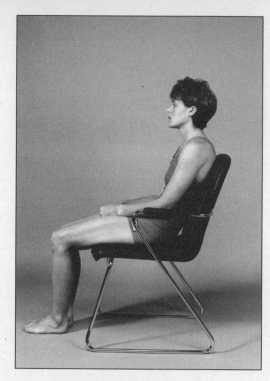

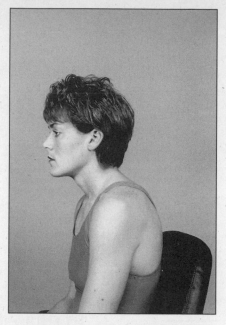

Figure 11.1a *Protruded head posture*

Figure 11.1 *Bad sitting posture*

When you sit, the position of the lower back strongly influences the posture of the neck. If the lower back is allowed to slouch, it is impossible to sit with the head and neck pulled backward. You can easily verify this for yourself. Unfortunately, once we have been sitting in a certain position for a few minutes, our body sags and we end up sitting slouched with a rounded lower back *and* a protruded head and neck. For most people, sitting for long periods results in sitting with poor posture.

Environmental Factors

The design of seating found in business and industrial settings, transportation, and the home only encourages poor postural habits. Rarely do the chairs and seats available give adequate support to the lower back and neck and, unless a conscious effort is made to sit correctly, we are forced to sit badly.

Case History: Behind the 8 Ball

Rikki is a 38-year-old factory worker in Michigan. For three months before beginning the McKenzie program, she had pain in the neck, left shoulder, and upper left arm. She said her neck pain was an 8 on a scale of zero to 10.

The pain would get worse during the day. In her job, she sat on a stool with no back. She had to lean over a bench and install small wires in electric motors. She had extremely poor posture, and her McKenzie-credentialed physical therapist performed a manual correction of the lumbar spine while Rikki was sitting. This immediately improved Rikki's posture and reduced her neck pain; the patient now said the level of pain was a 4.

The physical therapist introduced Rikki to the McKenzie exercises, in particular the "slouch-overcorrect" movements for posture and Neck Exercise 1, Head Retraction in Sitting. This exercise allowed Rikki to almost eliminate her arm and shoulder pain. Her neck pain centralized and declined to what she rated as a 3. At home, she continued with "slouch-overcorrect" and Neck Exercise 1, Head Retraction in Sitting.

In her second physical therapy visit, Rikki progressed to Neck Exercise 2, Neck Extension in Sitting. With her hands, she added "overpressure" to the exercise, resulting in greater extension. As a result of Neck Exercises 1 and 2, her symptoms were completely resolved. After six visits with the McKenzie therapist, Rikki was able to complete an eight-hour work day without any symptoms recurring. She remained on a home program of postural correction and neck exercise. As a result, she remained pain-free.

For the neck, ideally the back of the chair will come up high enough so that we can rest our head against it. But many seats provide no support for the head. An exception are the seats manufactured for most airlines, but, unfortunately, their head supports push the head and neck into the very same protruded position that causes our problems. It is the brave person indeed who takes the risk of sleeping in one of these seats, because when he or she wakes up he or she may well feel the old familiar pains in the neck.

When traveling by car, train, bus, or plane, we often are compelled to sit in the position dictated by the seats provided. It may be necessary for the driver of a car, bus, or truck to protrude the head and neck in order to see through the windshield; this is especially likely in bad weather.

Furniture in offices and factories all over the world is often designed poorly. Improvements have been made in the past decade, but not enough. And, to make matters worse, the furniture is rarely adaptable to individual requirements. This is one of the reasons that so many people who spend most of their day in a seated working position develop lower back and neck pain. Until all furniture designers understand the requirements of the human frame and begin to manufacture their chairs accordingly, we will continue to suffer from their neglect.

Finally, the design of domestic furniture is not any better. Unless your favorite living room chair is exceptional, you will have insufficient support in the lower back and the neck and will continue to place strains on these areas when you relax in the evening. If your neck problems are aggravated by reading or watching television, it is unlikely that the story is giving you a pain in the neck. The cause of the pain is not a ridiculous plot or unconvincing acting but rather the posture you have adopted. And this posture depends to a large extent on the type of chair or support you use.

Although the poor design of furniture contributes to the development of back problems, equal blame lies with the way we use the furniture. If we do not know how to sit correctly, even the best-designed chairs will not prevent us from slouching. On the other hand, once we are reeducated in correct sitting, bad chairs will not have a big impact on our posture.

How to Manage Prolonged Sitting Situations

In order to *prevent the development of neck pain* due to sitting poorly for long periods, you will need to (1) sit correctly and (2) interrupt the protruded-head posture or prolonged neck-bending at regular intervals.

In order to *treat neck pain* resulting from poor posture, you may need to perform other exercises in addition to correcting your posture. In this chapter I will discuss only the exercises required to reduce postural stresses and to correct your posture. The exercises for relief of pain and for increase of function will be described in the next chapter.

Correction of the Sitting Posture

You may have been sitting slouched for many years without neck and shoulder pain. But once you have developed neck problems, you must no longer sit in the old way, because the slouched posture will only continue the overstretching discussed previously.

If you are sitting slouched, with the lower back rounded, it is not possible to correct the posture of the neck (Fig. 11.2). Therefore you must *first correct the posture of your lower back*. Ideally, you will now review Chapter 4 of this book, Common Causes of Lower Back Pain, and especially its advice on how to improve your posture when you sit and stand.

For the purposes of this chapter, however, you must be fully aware of the following. The lumbar lordosis, the natural hollow present in your lower back when you stand, must be maintained during sitting in order for you to sit correctly (Fig. 11.3). To achieve this, *the use of a lumbar roll is essential*. A lumbar roll is a specially designed support for your lower back (Fig. 11.4). The roll should be no more than four to five inches (about 10–13 centimeters) in diameter before being compressed, and should be filled with foam of moderate density. Without this support, your lower back slouches and your head protrudes as soon as you relax or concentrate on anything other than your posture. Examples are when you talk,

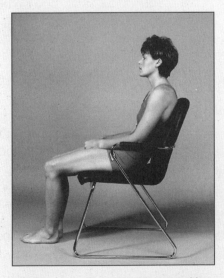

Figure 11.2 *Bad neck posture resulting from insufficient lower back support*

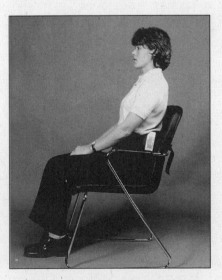

Figure 11.3 *Good neck posture made possible by use of a lumbar roll*

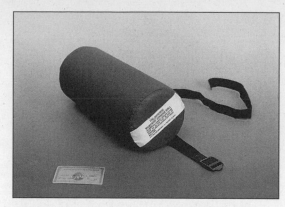

Figure 11.4 *Lumbar roll*

read, write, watch TV, and drive your car. To counteract this slouching, you must place the lumbar roll in the small of your back at the level of your beltline; you must do this whenever you sit in an easy chair (Fig. 11.5), car (Fig. 11.6), or office chair (Figs. 11.7 and 11.7a).

You may purchase a lumbar roll made specifically for the above purpose from the authorized firm listed in Appendix B of this book. You will need to supply your waist measurement and your weight.

In order to correct your neck's posture when you sit, you must first learn *how to retract your head*. Therefore you must become fully practiced in Exercise 1, Head Retraction in Sitting (see Chapter 12). You should perform this exercise 15 to 20 times per session, and you should perform the session three times per day, preferably morning, noon, and evening. The rhythmic procedure of the exercise (remember to slowly say "pressure on,

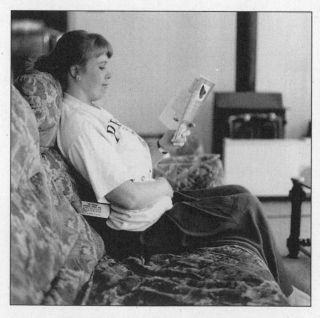

Figure 11.5 *A lumbar roll enables you to counteract slouching when you sit in an easy chair.*

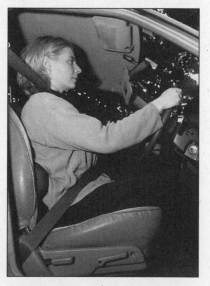

Figure 11.6 *Use of lumbar roll to correct poor car seat design*

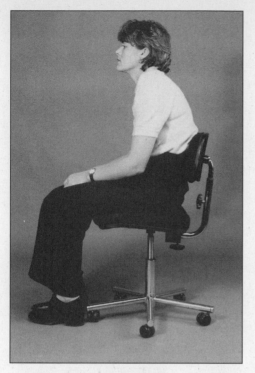

Figure 11.7
Poor office chair design uncorrected

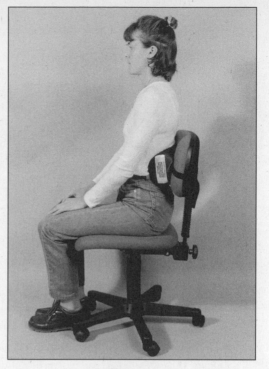

Figure 11.7a
Poor office chair design corrected by lumbar roll

pressure off"; see Chapter 4) teaches you the correct position of your head in relation to your body.

Each backward movement of the head must be performed to the maximum possible degree. When you have pulled your head back as far as possible, you have assumed the "retracted head posture" (Fig. 11.8). Now you have reached the extreme of the corrected head and neck posture.

Once you know how to retract your head, you must learn *how to find and maintain the correct head and neck posture*. The extreme of the retracted head position is a position of strain and it is not possible to sit this way for long. To sit comfortably and correctly, you must hold your head just short of the extreme retracted posture. To find this position, first retract the head as far as possible (Fig. 11.8), then release the last 10 percent of this movement (Fig. 11.9). Now you have reached the correct head and neck posture, which can be maintained for any length of time. It may take up to a week or so of practice to master this. The aim of this part of the program is to first restore the correct posture and then to maintain it.

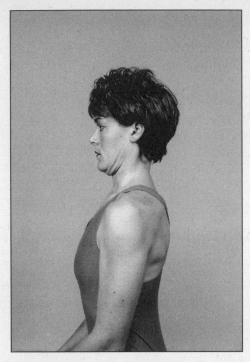

Figure 11.8 *"Retracted head posture"*

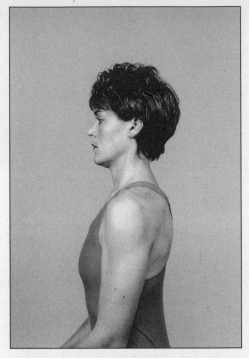

Figure 11.9 *After retracting the head, release the last 10 percent of movement.*

As a rule, the pain will decrease as your head posture improves, and you will have no pain once you maintain the correct posture. The pain will readily recur in the first few weeks whenever you allow your head to protrude. But eventually you will remain completely pain-free, even when you accidentally forget your posture.

Even so, you should never again allow yourself to sit for long periods in a slouched position with your head protruded. As soon as you have been completely pain-free for a couple of days, you can resume your normal activities. If from now on you follow the instructions in this book, you may also be able to prevent further neck trouble.

When you first use the above procedures to correct your lower back and neck posture in sitting, you will experience some new pains. These may differ from your original pain and may be felt in a new location. New pains are the result of performing new exercises and maintaining new positions. They should be expected and will wear off in a few days, provided postural correction is continued on a regular basis. Once you have become used to sitting correctly, you will enjoy it. You soon will notice the reduction or absence of pain and will experience an increased level of comfort. From then on, you will automatically choose chairs that allow you to sit correctly.

> RULE: When sitting for long periods, you must sit correctly, with the lower back supported by a lumbar roll and the head retracted.

Regular Interruption of Prolonged Neck Bending

If you spend long periods of time in the sitting position—for example, while working at a desk or knitting—it is likely that, even with the best intentions, you will eventually forget to maintain the correct posture. Gradually you will assume a more or less protruded head posture or a position in which both head and neck are bent forward. To counteract this, you must frequently interrupt the forward-bent position by correcting your neck posture and stretching your head and neck backward (see Exercise 2 in Chapter 12). This will relieve the stresses on the discs between the vertebrae as well as on the surrounding tissues.

> RULE: When sitting for long periods, it is essential to regularly interrupt prolonged bending of the neck. You can achieve this by retracting the head and extending the neck five or six times at regular intervals, for example once an hour.

2. LYING DOWN AND RESTING

Other than sitting, the most frequent cause of neck pain is postural stress in the lying position. If you wake up in the morning with a stiff and painful neck that was not causing problems the night before, there is likely to be something wrong with the surface on which you are lying or with the

Case History: What a Headache

Colleen, from Ohio, is a 27-year-old customer service agent with an airline. She had pain in the neck and the right shoulder blade. There was no known cause for the pain. The pain radiated down her right arm to her thumb and she had occasional headaches. When she started the McKenzie program, she had had these symptoms for about two months and they had gotten worse for three weeks. Activities that were painful included looking down, writing, being a passenger in a car, and turning her head, especially to the left. Her sleep was disturbed.

Colleen's neck's range of motion was limited. With McKenzie postural techniques, including use of a lumbar roll, her sitting posture improved and her neck and shoulder blade pain declined. Head Retraction in Sitting (Neck Exercise 1) reduced her symptoms and they remained better. She used a cervical roll for sleeping.

Four days after beginning the McKenzie program, Colleen had less neck pain and her headaches were less frequent and less intense. The cervical roll had enabled her to sleep without pain. Her range of motion had improved.

Three days later, the headaches were gone. Colleen noticed shoulder blade pain only when she woke up. She still had some pain when returning to a normal head position after looking down.

She began using the "slouch-overcorrect" technique to further improve her posture. Two weeks later Colleen was free of pain and had full range of motion.

position in which you are sleeping. It's a comparatively easy task to correct the surface on which you are lying, but rather difficult to influence the position you adopt while sleeping. Once you are asleep, you may just regularly change your position or you may toss and turn. Unless a certain position causes so much discomfort that it wakes you up, you have no real idea of the various positions you assume while sleeping.

Correction of Surface

All that is required to correct the surface on which you are lying is to use a different pillow. You may need to change the material, the thickness, or both. You must realize that the main function of the pillow is to *support both head and neck*. Therefore it should fill the natural hollow in the contour of the neck between the head and shoulder girdle without tilting the head or lifting it up. The head itself should be allowed to rest in a dish-shaped hollow.

It follows that you must easily be able to adjust the contents of the pillow. Ideally your pillow will be made of feathers, with a second choice being chips made of rubber or foam plastic.

By pulling and pushing the contents of the pillow, you can make a hollow for your neck and can bunch the edge to form a thick support for your neck. Pillows made of molded rubber or foam plastic do not allow their contents to be adjusted. They always adopt the shape of their original mold, regardless of attempts to change them. They do not permit the head to rest in a dish-shaped hollow but tend to apply a recoil pressure against the natural position the head would like to adopt. If you have such a pillow, you should replace it.

If your pillow is made of a recommended material but still does not provide adequate support for your neck, you should also use a supportive roll. A roll used for the neck is called a "cervical roll." Make a soft foam roll of about three inches (about eight centimeters) in diameter

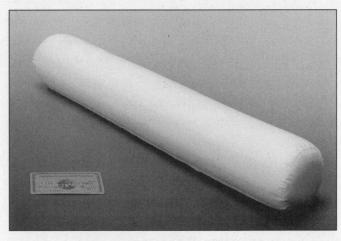

Figure 11.10   *Soft foam cervical roll...*

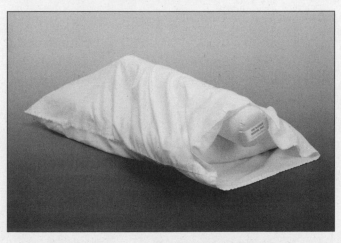

Figure 11.11   *...positioned inside a pillowcase...*

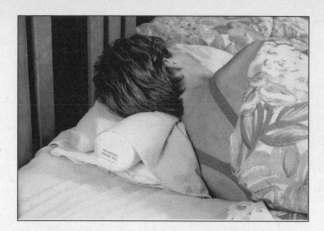

Figure 11.11a   . . . in order to support the neck.

and 18 inches (about 45 centimeters) long (Fig. 11.10). Place this inside your pillowcase, on top of the pillow and along its lower border (Fig. 11.11).

Alternatively, you can use a small hand towel of about 20 inches (about 50 centimeters) long and wide. Fold the towel in half and roll it loosely, then wind it around your neck and pin the ends together at the front. In both cases, the supportive roll will fill the space between the pillow and the neck (Fig. 11.11a). The measurements given above are merely a guide. All neck supports must fulfill individual requirements, and each person needs to experiment for himself or herself.

You may purchase a cervical roll made specifically for the above purpose from the authorized firm listed in Appendix B of this book. You will need to provide your neck measurement and your weight.

Correction of the Lying Posture

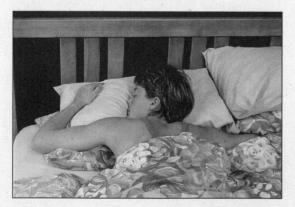

Figure 11.12
This sleeping position causes excessive strain.

If the lying posture itself is thought to cause neck pain, it needs to be investigated for each person individually, largely by trial and error. Consult a credentialed member or associate of the McKenzie Institute (see Appendix A). But there is one position that requires further discussion. Some people like to sleep lying facedown; many of these people frequently wake up with a pain in the neck or with a headache, which wears off as the day progresses. Other than this, they seem to have no neck problems.

While its owner is lying facedown, the head is usually turned to one side. In this position some of the joints, especially in the upper neck, reach the maximum possible degree of turning or come very close to it (Fig. 11.12). Consequently, this position places great strains on the soft tissues surrounding the joints of the neck and the soft tissues of the joints between the upper neck and the head.

If you sleep lying facedown and awake with pain in the neck or with a headache, you must avoid lying facedown. In addition, you should perform exercises for the neck, in particular Exercises 1, 2, and 6 (see Chapter 12). This is to ensure that you can retract the head and can extend the neck properly and that you have an adequate range of movement when turning the head.

3. RELAXING AFTER VIGOROUS ACTIVITY

When you have finished a vigorous activity—for example, playing football or tennis or chopping wood—and have not suffered any pain as a result, *you should not relax by sitting or lying with the head in a protruded posture* (Figs. 11.13 and 11.14). Thoroughly exercised spinal joints easily distort if they are held in an overstretched position for a long period. A commonly heard story is that when a person sits down to rest following demanding exercise or hard work, sometime later he or she has such severe pain that he or she can hardly move the neck. As with people who suffer back pain not long after playing a sport, usually people blame the exercise or work for their neck pain, but usually the pain has actually been produced by prolonged forward bending of the head and neck.

4. WORKING IN AWKWARD POSITIONS
OR CRAMPED SPACES

Some jobs can be performed only in positions that are likely to cause overstretching of the neck. These jobs may require you to sit, and usually

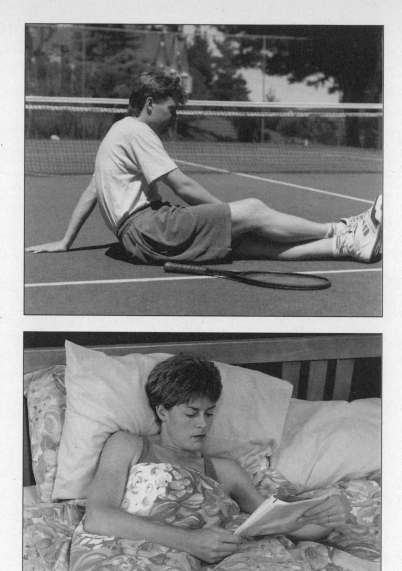

Figures 11.13–11.14
*After a vigorous activity, do not relax by sitting or lying with
the head in a protruded position.*

they involve precision work. Alternatively, they may have to be performed in cramped spaces or with the head and neck in awkward static (un-moving) positions. Under these circumstances, you may not be able to prevent the onset of neck pain just by regularly assuming the correct posture. If your neck problems are brought on by a job of the nature just described, you must, in addition to correcting your posture, frequently interrupt your overstretching and must perform Exercise 6 and Exercises 1 and 2 (see Chapter 12).

> RULE: When working with head and neck in a static position, interrupt this position at regular intervals by assuming the correct posture. In addition, perform five or six movements of Exercise 6, then Exercises 1 and 2 (see Chapter 12).

5. OSTEOPOROSIS

Beginning in middle age, many women are affected by osteoporosis. This is essentially a mineral-deficiency disorder. Although it affects the back more commonly than the neck, osteoporosis can cause symptoms in the neck as well.

For a more complete discussion of osteoporosis, see Chapter 8, Special Back Situations. In particular, see that chapter's discussion of the Mayo Clinic study that showed that extension exercises reduced the incidence of compression fractures in the back. One can infer from the Mayo study that people suffering from osteoporosis of the neck would reduce their incidence of pain and injury if they were to do the neck extension exercises described in this book. All of the neck exercises in this book except Neck Exercise 7 are extension exercises.

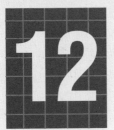

12 The McKenzie Method Exercises for the Neck

GENERAL GUIDELINES AND PRECAUTIONS

The McKenzie neck exercise program consists of seven exercises. The McKenzie *back* exercise program consists of seven different exercises; you will find them in Chapter 5.

Even though there are seven exercises, it is unlikely that in any one exercise session you will need to do more than two. So the exercise program is neither hard nor time-consuming.

The purposes of the McKenzie neck exercises are to eliminate pain and, where possible, to restore normal function; that is, to regain full mobility in the neck or as much movement as is possible under the given circumstances. When you are exercising for pain relief, you should move to the edge of the pain or just into the pain, then release the pressure and return to the starting position. But when you are exercising for stiffness, the exercises can be made more effective by using your hands and gently but firmly applying overpressure (more pressure than you can apply just through unassisted movement of the head or neck) in order to obtain the maximum amount of movement. After doing the exercises, you should always correct your posture and then maintain the correct posture. Once you no longer have neck pain, good postural habits will be essential to prevent the recurrence of neck problems.

In order to determine whether the exercise program in this chapter is right for you, it is very important that you observe closely any changes in the location of the pain. You may notice that, as a result of the exercises, the pain, originally felt on one side of the spine, across the shoulders, or down the arm, moves toward the center of your neck. In other words, your pain localizes or centralizes. *As with back pain, centralization of neck pain (Fig. 12.1) that takes place as you exercise is a good sign.* If your pain moves from areas farther away from the neck—that is, if it moves from areas in which it usually is felt—and toward the midline of the spine, that means

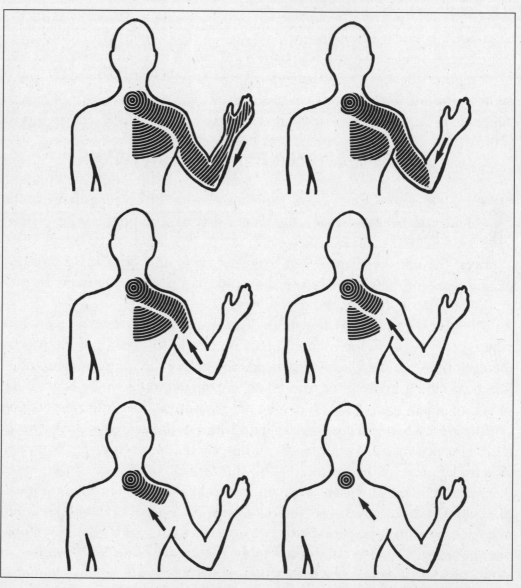

Figure 12.1   *The progressive centralization of pain as a result of the McKenzie exercise program*

you are exercising correctly and that the McKenzie exercise program is the right one for you.

If your neck pain is so intense that you can move your head only with difficulty and cannot find a position that permits you to lie in bed comfortably, your approach to the exercises should be especially cautious and unhurried.

On beginning any of the exercises, you may notice an increase in pain. *This initial pain increase is common and can be expected.* As you continue to practice the exercises, the pain should quickly diminish, at least to the level you experienced before the exercises. Usually this occurs during the first exercise session. This should then be followed by centralization of pain.

Once the pain no longer spreads outward and once it is felt only at the midline, the intensity of pain will decrease rapidly over a period of two to three days. In another two to three days, your pain should disappear entirely.

In summary and addition, pain can improve in many ways:

- It can become less intense.

- It can become less frequent.

- You can sustain activity longer before the pain occurs.

- You can move farther before pain begins.

- Constant pain can be replaced by intermittent pain.

- Pain can centralize. (This not only provides for a more comfortable type of pain but predicts a good outcome through the McKenzie exercises.)

If, however, following an initial increase in pain, the pain continues to increase or spreads to places farther away from the spine, immediately stop exercising. Seek advice from a health professional. In other words, do not continue with any of the exercises if your symptoms are much worse immediately after exercising and remain worse the next day. Also stop the exercises if, during exercise, you experience symptoms in the arm below the elbow for the first time or if you experience a worsening in symptoms below the elbow that you already had.

If you need advice from a health professional, ideally you will consult a credentialed member or associate of the McKenzie Institute. To obtain the names of these practitioners, see Appendix A at the back of this book.

If your symptoms have been present more or less continuously for many weeks or months, you should not expect to be pain-free in two or three days. The response will be slower than if your symptoms were recent, but if you are doing the correct exercises, it will be only a matter of 10 to 14 days before the pain subsides. If you are lucky, it will be faster than that.

When learning the exercises, you should adopt the sitting position. Once you fully master them, you may exercise while sitting or standing, whichever you prefer.

Nevertheless, if the pain is too acute for you to tolerate the exercises while sitting, you may need to begin exercising while lying down. In the lying position, the pain will be reduced, because the head and neck are better supported and the compressive forces on the spine are considerably less. If you are age 60 or older, it is also advisable to begin exercising while lying down. People of older age groups occasionally experience dizziness or light-headedness when performing extension exercises involving the head (of the seven exercises in this chapter, Exercises 1–6 all involve extension). If symptoms such as these persist, stop the exercises and seek advice from a health professional. On the other hand, when the initial attempts at extension exercises in lying do not have any ill effects, you can safely proceed to exercising while sitting.

If, due to a medical problem, it is difficult or not advisable for you to lie flat, you should restrict yourself to exercising in the sitting position. People who are over 60 and who also should not lie flat should attempt the exercises from a sitting position but should be cautious when first trying them. The first time they try the exercise, they should have another person at their side to assist in the event of dizziness or light-headedness.

When beginning this exercise program, you should stop any other exercises that you may have been shown by a health professional. You should also temporarily stop any workout or sports activities. If you want to continue with exercises other than those described in this book, you should wait until your pains have completely subsided. If you are intent on returning to sports before your pain has subsided, you must nonetheless avoid all contact sports. As for non-contact sports, you can gently attempt a return to them; if, after a short trial, your pain is worse, you must discontinue even non-contact sports until your pains have completely subsided.

Once you have started this exercise program, new pains may develop, because you are performing movements your body is not used to. The new pains are different from your original pain and are usually felt in areas of the neck and shoulder girdle that were not previously affected. But, provided you continue with the exercises, these pains will wear off in three to four days.

I always suspect that if my patients have not complained of new pains, they have not been exercising adequately or they have not been putting enough effort into correcting their posture. Both new exercises and new postures are likely to cause temporary new pains.

I cannot overstress the importance of doing the exercises precisely as they are described in this book. That is, it is important to do each exercise exactly as it is described and to do the exercises in the order that is set out in this book. The failure to heed even one sentence in the description of an exercise can keep the exercise from being effective. Don't figure that you can save time by glancing at the instructions for a particular exercise or by trying to learn an exercise just by looking at the photographs that accompany it. In this way you may save a minute or two, but may slow your recovery by weeks—not a good bargain.

Similarly, don't skimp. Generally, the exercises should be done six to eight times a day. If you do them once or twice a day, you may gain some benefit, but not nearly what you would gain if you did them as often as prescribed.

There are decades of clinical experience and research behind these exercises: how to do them, in what order to do them, how often to do them. I want you to benefit as much as possible from them. Don't get in the way of your own recovery!

NECK EXERCISE 1
Head Retraction in Sitting

This is the first McKenzie exercise for the *neck*. Again, if you are a *back* patient, you will find the McKenzie exercises for the back in Chapter 5.

Head retraction means pulling the head backward.

Sit on a chair or stool, look straight ahead, and allow yourself to relax completely. As you do this, your head will protrude a little (Fig. 12.2). Now you are ready to start the first and most important exercise.

Move your head slowly but steadily backward until it is pulled back as far as you can manage (Fig. 12.3). As you do this, it is important to *keep your chin tucked down and in.* In other words, you must remain looking straight ahead and should not tilt the head backward as in looking up. When your head is pulled back as far as possible, you have assumed the retracted head posture (Fig. 12.3). Once you have maintained this position for a few seconds, you should relax, and automatically your head and neck will protrude again (Fig. 12.2). Each time you repeat this cycle of movements, you must make sure that the backward movement of the head and neck is performed to the *maximum possible degree.*

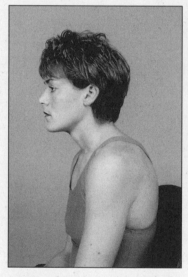

Figure 12.2 *The relaxed position allows the head to protrude.*

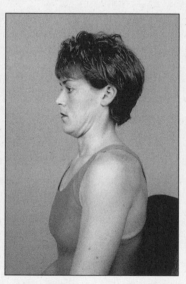

Figure 12.3 *The retracted position*

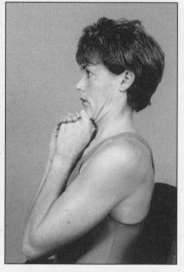

Figure 12.4 *Retraction with overpressure*

As with all other McKenzie Method neck and back exercises involving multiple movements, remember to slowly think or say the words "pressure on, pressure off," as you do the exercise. This helps you to hold each position just long enough and establishes a rhythm in which to do the exercise.

The exercise can be made more effective by placing both hands on the chin and firmly pushing the head even farther back (Fig. 12.4).

Case History: A Real (Estate) Story

Carl, 45, is a real estate agent in Massachusetts. Following an auto accident, he had sharp neck pain. He saw his chiropractor, and the appointments made his neck feel better but had no lasting effect.

Carl canceled all but his most critical appointments and rested at home as much as he could. One Saturday, his mother was to host a birthday party for Carl's younger brother, Dave. Carl didn't want to be the only absentee, so, with difficulty, he got himself to the restaurant where the party was being held. Dave told him how he himself had been helped by the McKenzie neck exercises. Even so, both Dave and Carl feared that Carl's pain was so sharp that it wouldn't respond to the exercises.

Nonetheless, the day after the party, Dave sent Carl a copy of the McKenzie neck exercises. Carl tried several of them. To his amazement, he found that just one of them—Exercise 1, Head Retraction in Sitting—gave him dramatic relief in just one session.

He continued with Exercise 1, added Exercise 2 (Neck Extension in Sitting), and paid careful attention to his posture. Within one week he was 80 percent better and two weeks later he was pain-free. His symptoms did not return.

This exercise is used mainly in the *treatment* of neck pain, as opposed to its *prevention*. When used in the *treatment* of neck pain, the exercise should be repeated 10 times per session, and the sessions should be spread evenly six to eight times throughout the day. This means you should repeat the sessions about every two hours. If you experience acute pains on attempting this exercise, you must replace it with Exercise 3, Head Retraction in Lying. When used in the *prevention* of neck pain, the exercise should be repeated five or six times as many times a day as required. That is, if you find you can prevent neck pain by performing two sessions of this exercise, then do two sessions a day, and if you can prevent it only by doing ten sessions a day, do ten.

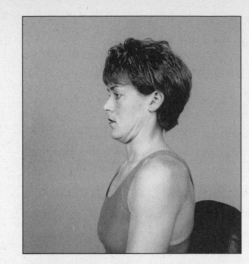

Figure 12.5   *The retracted position*

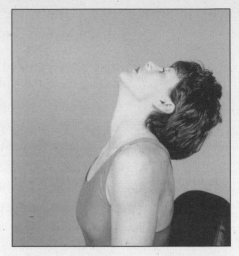

Figure 12.6   *Lift your chin up and tilt your head backward, as if you were looking up at the sky.*

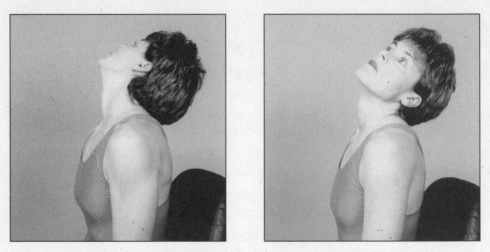

Figures 12.7–12.7a   *With your head tilted as far back as possible, repeatedly turn your nose just half an inch to the right and then to the left of the midline.*

NECK EXERCISE 2
Neck Extension in Sitting

Extension means bending backward.

This exercise should always follow Exercise 1. Remain seated, repeat Exercise 1 a few times, then hold your head in the retracted position (Fig. 12.5). Now you are ready to start Exercise 2.

Case History: Watch Out for Five-Year-Olds

Ronnie, a Californian, plays lead guitar in a well-known rock band. He is 52. Due to an auto accident whiplash injury, he had a recurring neck condition that most of the time caused him no pain. Two physical therapists who had treated him had shown him the McKenzie exercises. One evening he was standing near his five-year-old daughter. She expressed her affection by giving him a hug. Unfortunately, she chose to do this by jumping up and grabbing him around the neck, briefly suspending her 45 pounds from that fragile body part.

The guitar player had immediate pain. That evening he tried the McKenzie exercises as he remembered them, plus rest, ibuprofen, and ice. All helped some, none helped enough.

The next day he went to his office, where he had a copy of the McKenzie exercises. He realized that he had forgotten all about Exercise 2, Neck Extension in Sitting. He marveled at how the small point of moving the head left and right about a half-inch from the midline permitted him to make his head go back farther and farther.

In the first session of this exercise, Ronnie's pain was 70 percent better. He had improved so much that he could return to all his normal activities. The next session brought the improvement to about 80 percent. The next day, he was about 90 percent better. All due to one exercise and to doing it *exactly* as McKenzie instructs patients to do it. Within two weeks, his symptoms were entirely gone.

Lift your chin up and tilt your head backward, as if you were looking up at the sky (Fig. 12.6). As you do this, *do not allow your neck to move forward.* With your head tilted back as far as possible, repeatedly turn your nose just half an inch (about two centimeters) to the right and then to the left of the midline (Figs. 12.7 and 12.7a), all the time attempting to move your head and neck even farther backward. Once you have done this for a few seconds, return your head to the starting position. Again, each time you repeat this cycle of movements, make sure your neck is extended as far as possible.

This exercise can be used both in the treatment and prevention of neck pain. Exercise 2 is to be performed 10 times per session, and the sessions should be spread evenly six to eight times throughout the day. If your pain is too acute to tolerate Exercise 2, you should replace it with Exercise 3, Head Retraction in Lying.

Once you are fully practiced in Exercises 1 and 2 separately from one another, you can combine these two exercises successfully into one exercise.

NECK EXERCISE 3
Head Retraction in Lying

Lie on a bed. Lie face up, with your head at a free-standing edge of the bed rather than next to any headboard. For example, lie across a double bed or with your head at the foot of a single bed. Rest your head and shoulders flat on the bed and do not use a pillow (Fig. 12.8). Now you are ready to start Exercise 3.

Using your head alone, not your hands, push the back of your head into the mattress and at the same time pull in your chin (Fig. 12.9). The overall effect should be that your head and neck move backward as far as possible while you keep facing the ceiling. Once you have maintained this position for a few seconds, relax. Automatically, your head and neck will return to the starting position (Fig. 12.8). Each time you repeat this cycle of movements, make sure that the backward movement of your head and neck is carried out to the maximum possible degree.

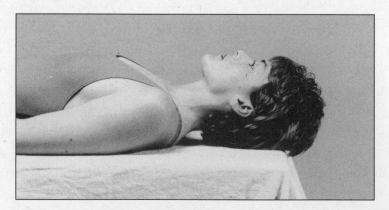

Figure 12.8
Rest your head and shoulders flat on the bed.

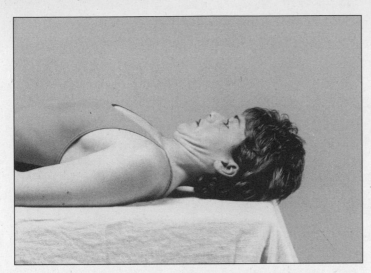

Figure 12.9 *Push the back of your head into the mattress and at the same time pull in your chin.*

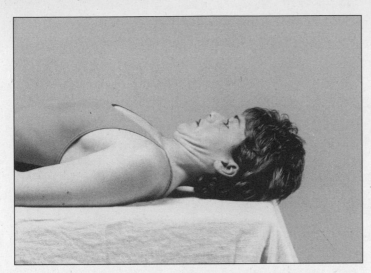

This exercise is used mainly in the treatment of acute neck pain. It is used mostly by people who have gained no benefit from exercises done in the sitting or standing position. It is an effective exercise, but not as demanding as most of the others. When you have completed 10 head retractions, you must evaluate the effects of this exercise on your pain. If the pain has centralized or decreased in intensity, you can safely continue this procedure. In this case you should repeat the exercise 10 times per session and spread the sessions evenly six to eight times throughout the day or night. (Since you already are in bed at night, night is a good time to repeat this exercise.)

If, however, the pain has increased considerably or extends farther away from the spine, or if you have developed "pins and needles," or numbness, in the fingers, you must stop the exercise and seek advice from a health professional. To locate a practitioner who is a credentialed member or associate of the McKenzie Institute, see Appendix A of this book.

NECK EXERCISE 4
Neck Extension in Lying

This exercise should always follow Exercise 3. You must again lie on the bed, face up. Before you can start Exercise 4, you must support your head by placing one hand under it. Now move up along the bed until your head, your neck, and the top of your shoulders are extended over the edge (Fig. 12.10).

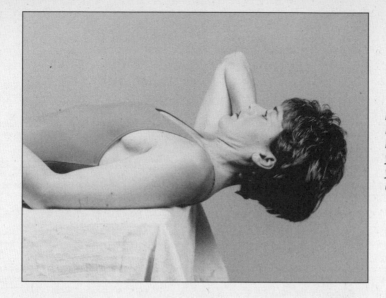

Figure 12.10
Place one hand under your head and extend your head, your neck, and the top of your shoulders over the edge of the bed.

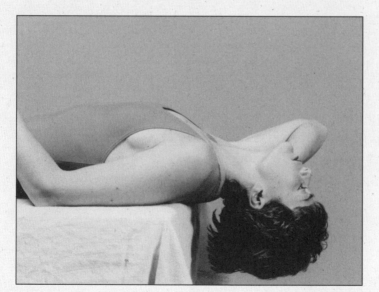

Figure 12.11
While supporting your head, lower it slowly toward the floor.

While continuing to support your head with your hand, lower your head slowly toward the floor (Fig. 12.11). Now, gradually remove your hand (Fig. 12.12) and bring your head and neck as far backward as you can, so that you can see as much as possible of the floor directly under you. In this position, repeatedly turn your nose just half an inch (about two cen-

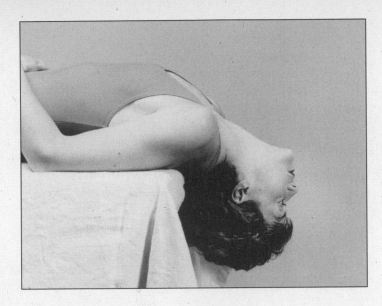

Figure 12.12
Gradually remove your hand and bring your head and neck as far backward as you can.

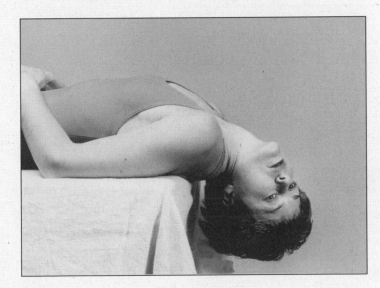

Figure 12.13
Repeatedly turn your nose just half an inch to the right and then to the left of the midline.

timeters) to the right and then to the left of the midline (Fig. 12.13), all the time attempting to move your head and neck farther backward. Once you have reached the maximum amount of extension, try to relax in this position for two to three seconds.

In order to return to the resting position, first place one hand behind your head, then help your head back to the horizontal position and move your body down along the bed until your head is lying fully on the bed again. It is important that, following this exercise, *you do not get up from the bed immediately* but that instead you rest for a few minutes with your head flat on the bed. *Do not use a pillow.*

As with Exercise 3, this exercise is used mainly in the treatment of acute neck pain. Also as with Exercise 3, it is effective, yet not as demanding as most of the others. Until the acute symptoms have subsided, Exercise 4 is to follow Exercise 3, and Exercise 4 should be done only once per session. Once you no longer have acute pains, Exercises 3 and 4 should be replaced by Exercises 1 and 2. By now you will have noticed that, except for the position in which they are performed, Exercises 3 and 4 are really the same as Exercises 1 and 2.

NECK EXERCISE 5
Sidebending of the Neck

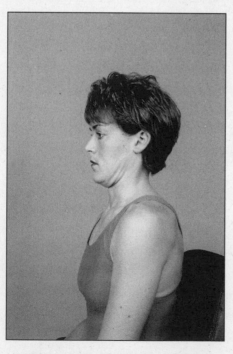

Figure 12.14 *The retracted position*

Sit on a chair. Repeat Exercise 1 a few times, then hold your head in the retracted position (Fig. 12.14). Now you are ready to start Exercise 5.

Bend your neck sideways and move your head toward the side on which you feel most of the pain. Do not allow the head to turn (Fig. 12.15). In other words, keep looking straight ahead and bring your ear—*not your nose*—close to your shoulder. It is important that you *keep the head well retracted as you do this. The exercise can be made more effective by using the hand of the painful side, placing it over the top of your head, and gently but firmly pulling your head even farther toward the painful side* (Fig. 12.16).

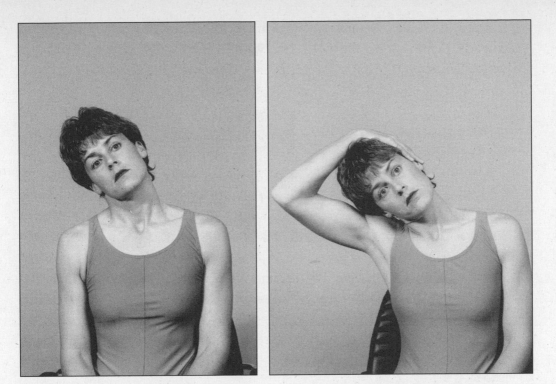

Figure 12.15 *Bend your neck sideways and move your head toward the side on which you feel most of the pain.*

Figure 12.16 *Gently but firmly pull your head even farther toward the painful side.*

Once you have maintained this position for a few seconds, return your head to the starting position.

This exercise is used specifically for the treatment of pain felt only to one side or pain felt much more to one side than the other. Until your symptoms have centralized, Exercise 5 is to be repeated 10 times per session and the sessions are to be spread evenly six to eight times throughout the day.

NECK EXERCISE 6
Neck Rotation

In this book, *rotation* means turning to the right and left.

Sit on a chair, repeat Exercise 1 a few times, then hold your head in the retracted position (Fig. 12.17). Now you are ready to start Exercise 6.

Turn your head far to the right and then far to the left, as though you

Case History: If at First You Don't Succeed . . .

Larry, a 48-year-old public interest lawyer in Washington, D.C., presents an example of a neck sufferer who at first did not benefit much from the exercises but then made a key adaptation. He suffered a whiplash injury when he was waiting to turn left at an intersection and a driver behind him was talking to her child instead of watching the road.

Larry's pain was chiefly on the right side, including not just the neck but the shoulder and upper back. Sometimes he had tingling in the fingers of his right hand. He saw his family doctor, then an orthopedist, and then a physical therapist for six months. He improved, but only slowly. Advil helped, but did nothing for the underlying cause of the pain.

Then Larry got a copy of the McKenzie exercises for the neck. Naturally enough, he started out with Neck Exercise 1, Head Retraction in Sitting, and Neck Exercise 2, Neck Extension in Sitting. These gave him only minor relief. But then he tried Neck Exercise 5, Sidebending of the Neck, which is indicated specifically for people with pain exclusively on one side or much more on one side than the other.

He improved rapidly. The first time he did the exercises, the pain centralized, and Larry found the pain much more tolerable in the central position than when it was on the right side. At the same time, the pain declined markedly. Within a week, the pain was no longer a problem in his life, and in about a month his symptoms had vanished entirely.

were about to cross a street (Fig. 12.18). As you do this, it is important that you *keep the head well retracted*. If you experience more pain as you turn to one side than to the other, continue the exercise by rotating only to the *more* painful side. As you repeatedly turn to that side, the pain should gradually centralize or decrease.

But if the pain increases and fails to centralize, continue the exercise by rotating only to the *less* painful side.

Once you have the same amount of pain when turning to either side, or have no pain when turning to either side, continue the exercise by rotating to both sides.

The exercise can be made more effective by using both hands and

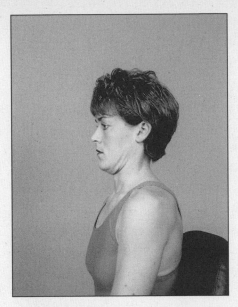

Figure 12.17 *The retracted position*

gently but firmly pushing your head even farther into rotation (Figs. 12.19 and 12.19a). Once you have maintained the position of maximum rotation for a few seconds, return your head to the starting position.

This exercise can be used in the treatment of neck pain as well as for its prevention. When used in the *treatment* of pain or stiffness of the neck, the exercise is to be performed 10 times per session, and the sessions are to be spread evenly six to eight times throughout the day. Whether or not centralization or a decrease in pain has taken place, *Exercise 6 must always be followed by Exercises 1 and 2.* When used in the *prevention* of neck problems, the exercise should be repeated five or six times every two or three days or as often as required.

NECK EXERCISE 7
Neck Flexion in Sitting

Flexion means bending forward.

Sit on a chair, look straight ahead, and allow yourself to relax completely (Fig. 12.20). Now you are ready to start Exercise 7.

Drop your head forward and let it rest with your chin as close as possible to your chest (Fig. 12.21). Place your hands behind the back of your head and interlock your fingers (Fig. 12.22). Now let your arms relax so that your

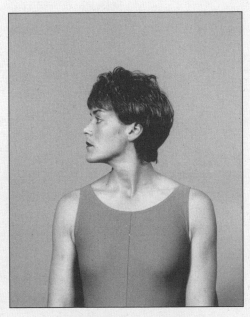

Figure 12.18 *Turn your head far to the right and then far to the left.*

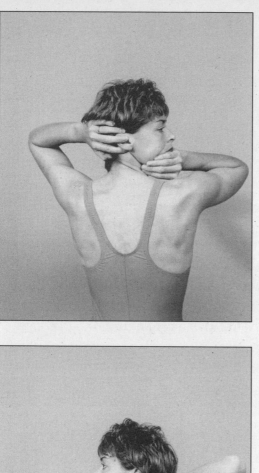

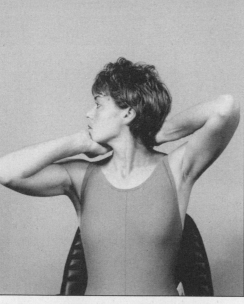

Figures 12.19–12.19a
Use both hands and gently but firmly push
your head even farther into rotation.

elbows point down toward the floor. In this position, the weight of your arms will pull your head down farther and bring your chin closer to your chest (Fig. 12.23).

This exercise can be made more effective by using your hands and gently but firmly pulling your head onto your chest. Once you have maintained the position of maximum neck flexion for a few seconds, return your head to the starting position.

This exercise is used mainly for the treatment of *headaches*, but can also be applied to resolve residual neck pain or stiffness once the acute symptoms have subsided. In both cases, it should be repeated only two or three times per session, and the sessions should be spread evenly six to eight times throughout the day.

When used in the treatment of headaches, Exercise 7 should be performed in conjunction with Exercise 1. For more on using the exercises when you have headaches, see the section When You Have Headaches, on page 178. When used in the treatment of neck pain or stiffness, Exercise 7 must always be followed by Exercises 1 and 2.

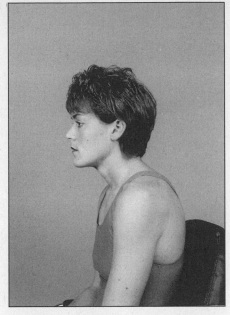

Figure 12.20
Sit on a chair, look straight ahead,
and allow yourself to relax completely.

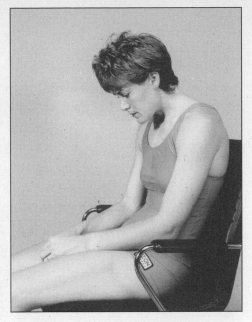

Figure 12.21   Drop your head forward and
let it rest with your chin as close as
possible to your chest.

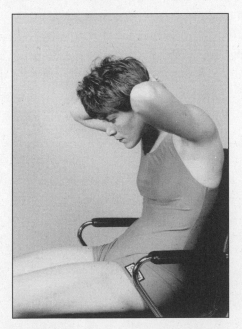

Figure 12.22   Place your hands behind the
back of your head and interlock your
fingers.

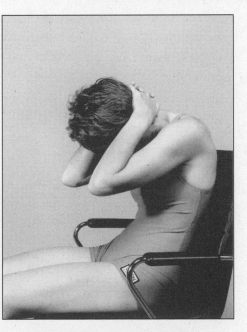

Figure 12.23   Let your arms relax so
the elbows point down toward the floor.

Case History: Convincing the Docs

Catherine lives in Arkansas. She is 40 years old and works as a receptionist in the office of several physicians. Before starting the McKenzie program, she had for four months suffered from neck pain, headaches, and difficulty in swallowing. Two months before the symptoms began, the medical office had been remodeled and she had been given a new phone system and a different desk.

Catherine's McKenzie-certified physical therapist concluded that Catherine had cervical disc inflammation resulting from her posture while talking on the phone and while typing on a computer keyboard; both these postures had changed because of the remodeling of the office.

The physical therapist prescribed Neck Exercise 7, Neck Flexion in Sitting. Doctors had attributed her swallowing difficulties to allergies, but with Neck Exercise 7, this symptom immediately disappeared. Before trying Exercise 7, Catherine reported pain at 5 on a 0–10 scale, but after doing Exercise 7 for the first time, she said her pain had declined to a 1.

Catherine visited the physical therapist four times over two weeks and threw away her allergy medications. Over this period, her neck pain and headaches resolved completely. She remained pain-free. She was not the only one impressed by the effects of the McKenzie program: after she reported her results to the people at her office, the physicians and co-workers also became believers in the McKenzie Method.

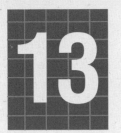

13 When to Do the Neck Exercises

WHEN YOU ARE IN SIGNIFICANT PAIN

Even if your pain is very acute, you may be able to get out of bed, although probably with difficulty. But certain movements will be impossible and often you will not be able to find a comfortable position in which to sit or work. Even though you are in acute pain, you should always attempt to begin with Exercise 1. Many people find that this exercise gives substantial relief from pain and that they do not have to start with the exercises that involve lying on a bed (Exercises 3 and 4).

As soon as possible, even on the first day, you should add Exercise 2. You should continue Exercises 1 and 2 until you feel considerably better. Once you no longer have acute pain, you should follow the exercise program as outlined in this chapter under the heading When Acute Pain Has Subsided.

If you have done three or four sessions of Exercise 1, spread over a period of 15 minutes, and the pain remains too acute to tolerate that exercise, you should stop it and replace it with Exercise 3. Your symptoms should gradually decrease and centralize so that there is some improvement by the time you have completed a few sessions. Exercise 4 should be added as soon as you have become well practiced in Exercise 3 and your symptoms have improved to some extent, or when Exercise 3 is no longer bringing you any improvement.

When the person with neck pain should introduce Exercise 4 varies from person to person, but the sooner you can do this, the better. It is important that you carefully watch the pain pattern. You are exercising correctly if in a few days the pain moves toward the base or the center of the neck and decreases. In time the pain should disappear entirely and be replaced by a feeling of strain or stiffness, a feeling that is more tolerable.

When you have improved significantly—usually two to three days after you began the exercises that involve lying on a bed, possibly earlier—you may gradually reduce the number of sessions of Exercises 3 and 4. As you do this, you should gradually introduce Exercises 1 and 2 and then gradually increase these two exercises.

In another few days you will be doing only exercises in sitting (instead of exercises done while lying on a bed), and you will find that they give you the same pain relief as you previously obtained by exercising while on a bed. At this stage, the periods that you are completely free of pain are becoming more frequent and are beginning to last longer.

Again, once you feel considerably better and no longer have acute pain, you should continue the exercise program as outlined for when acute pain has subsided. (That program is set out under When Acute Pain Has Subsided.)

NO RESPONSE OR BENEFIT

When pain is felt only to one side of the spine or much more to one side than the other, the exercises recommended so far sometimes fail to bring relief. If this is the case, you should begin with Exercise 5. Whether or not centralization or decrease in pain has taken place, Exercise 5 must always be followed by Exercises 1 and 2. After two or three days of practice, you may notice that the pain is distributed more evenly across the spine or has centralized. Once either of these events has occurred, you may gradually reduce Exercise 5.

When you are considerably better and the pain has fully centralized, you should continue with the exercise program as outlined for when acute pain has subsided. (See right.)

WHEN ACUTE PAIN HAS SUBSIDED

Once the acute pain has passed, you may still feel some pain or stiffness when you move in certain ways. You will notice this most clearly when you turn your neck to one side or the other or when you bend your head and neck forward in order to look down. It is likely that at this stage, healing of overstretched or damaged soft tissues has taken place. Now you must ensure that the elasticity of these soft tissues and the flexibility of your spine as a whole are restored without causing you further damage.

If you have pain on turning your head to the right or left, you should practice Exercise 6. If you have pain on bending your head forward, you need to practice Exercise 7. Each time you repeat an exercise, you must move to the edge of the pain and then release the pressure. The pain should disappear entirely over a period of two to three weeks. Each session of Exercises 6 and 7 should always be concluded with a few repetitions of Exercises 1 and 2.

If you feel stiffness but no pain in these exercises, you should do the same exercises but apply overpressure with your hands at the end of each movement. By exercising in this way, you achieve the maximum possible movement. In three to six weeks you should be able to restore normal function.

Once you are completely symptom-free, you should follow the guidelines given to prevent recurrence of neck problems, found under When You Have No Pain or Stiffness, which follows immediately.

WHEN YOU HAVE NO PAIN OR STIFFNESS

Many people with neck problems have lengthy spells in which they experience little or no pain. If, in the past or recently, you have had one or more episodes of neck pain, you should start the exercise program even though at the moment you may be pain-free. Nevertheless, in this situation it is not necessary to do all the exercises you would do if you were in pain or to exercise every two hours.

To prevent recurrence of neck problems, you should do Exercise 6, followed by Exercises 1 and 2. You should do these regularly, preferably in the morning and at night. Furthermore, whenever you feel minor strain developing during work or while sitting, you should do Exercises 1 and 2. It is even more important that you watch your posture at all times and never again let postural stresses cause you neck pain.

These exercises will have very little or no effect if you constantly fall back into poor posture. It may be necessary to exercise in the manner described above for the rest of your life, but it is essential that you develop and maintain good postural habits.

As it takes only one minute to perform one session of Exercise 6 and another minute to combine Exercises 1 and 2 and repeat them 10 times, lack of time should never be used as an excuse for not doing the exercises.

RECURRENCE

At the first sign of recurrence of neck pain, you should immediately perform Exercises 1 and 2. If your pain already is too acute to tolerate these exercises, or if they fail to reduce your pain, you must quickly introduce Exercises 3 and 4. If you have one-sided symptoms that do not centralize with any of these exercises, you should start with Exercise 5. Again, you must pay extra attention to your posture, regularly perform postural correction, and maintain the correct posture as much as you can.

WHEN YOU HAVE HEADACHES

Headaches often can be relieved by some of the recommended exercises, usually Exercises 1 and 7. Unless your neck pain is severe, it will not do any harm to perform these exercises for a couple of days in order to find out whether you benefit from them or not. In the first three days, you should perform Exercise 1, Head Retraction in Sitting, at regular intervals and whenever you feel a headache is developing. If this reduces your headaches but does not eliminate them, you should add Exercise 7. Exercise 7 is particularly effective in relieving headaches that spread over the top of your head to above or behind the eyes. You may even be able to *prevent* such headaches by performing this exercise as soon as you feel minor strain building up.

In case your headaches are not relieved by these two exercises, for the next three days you should do Exercise 4, Neck Extension in Lying, followed by Exercises 1 and 2 and postural correction. As your symptoms improve, you may gradually stop Exercise 4 but you must continue Exercises 1 and 2.

If you are unable to influence your headaches with any of the exercises or if your headaches become much worse during exercising and remain worse over the next day, you should stop exercising and seek advice from a health professional. A credentialed member or associate of the McKenzie Institute would be especially well qualified to assist you. To obtain the names of these practitioners, see Appendix A at the back of this book.

14 Instructions for People with Acute Neck Pain

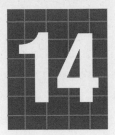

Chances are that you can use this book immediately. Nevertheless, if you have developed neck pain for the first time and it is no better 10 days after onset, do not use this book until you have consulted your doctor. Also, if you have complications to your neck problems, do not use this book until you have consulted the same person. Examples of complications are severe, stabbing pains, or that your head is pulled off-center, or that you have severe, continuing headaches.

Keep your head up at all times. When you allow the head to droop while you are engaged in activities such as working at a desk, reading, knitting, or sewing, you place further strains on the already overstretched or injured tissues. It is essential to maintain good posture.

Do not roll your head around. Avoid quick movements, especially turning the head quickly.

Avoid the positions and movements that caused your problems in the first place. You must allow some time for healing to take place.

Do not sleep with more pillows than necessary. If you are comfortable with one pillow, then use only one. The contents of the pillow should be adjustable so that the pillow provides proper support for the neck.

When you remain uncomfortable while sleeping or attempting to sleep, you may benefit by placing a cervical roll inside your pillowcase.

Do not sleep facedown, as this places great strains on the neck.

Do not lie in the bath for any length of time, as this bends your head and neck forward, excessively.

Carefully start the self-treatment exercises. Remember, an initial increase in pain can be expected when beginning any of the exercises. This pain should decrease or centralize, or both, as you repeat the movements.

(In the event that you have a sudden onset of acute neck pain and need a quick summary of what to do, consult Chapter 16, Panic Pages for the Neck, which starts on page 189.)

ALTERNATIVES TO EXERCISE

Health professionals and others offer many ways to treat neck pain. In Chapter 9, I deal with many of these, regarding how they relate to back pain. Because the way health professionals treat back pain has much in common with how they treat neck pain, most of what I say in Chapter 9 also applies to what I could say about the alternatives that these professionals provide. Therefore I refer you to Chapter 9. Chapter 9 deals with medicines and drugs, bed rest, acupuncture, chiropractic, and electrotherapy (heat, shortwave diathermy, and ultrasound). I also discuss back pain in the community.

With few exceptions, I would simply substitute the word "neck" for "back" and "lower back" and then leave Chapter 9 as is. One exception is that bed rest, while appropriate in a small minority of cases of back pain, is appropriate even more rarely for neck pain. While a bed may be the only practical way to support a severely painful back, a much smaller device supports the neck fairly well in those cases where the neck should be treated almost exclusively by resting it. In these rare cases you should consult a doctor and then, if he or she recommends doing so, give your neck a rest by using a soft foam rubber cervical collar for short periods. Continue to use it if it immediately reduces your discomfort, but do not use it for more than three or four weeks.

Regarding neck pain in the community, a difference between Chapter 9 and what I would say about the neck is that in Western countries, approximately 40 percent will at one time suffer a severe neck pain episode (not the 80 percent in the case of the back).

Because the neck depends on good back posture, the neck patient, just like the back patient, should seek good furniture and good seating in transit situations and should complain when these are not available. Similarly, it is important not only for the back but the neck that school physical education instructors teach posture and the consequences of bad posture. Again, for information on the McKenzie Institute Postural Video, which is available to schools, please see Appendix A.

Panic Pages for the Back

In case of a sudden onset of acute back pain, observe the following precautions. Then, if you can use this book, proceed with the instructions.

PRECAUTIONS

If you have unusual complications, do not use this book or this chapter until you have consulted your doctor, physical therapist, or chiropractor. These complications include constant pain that travels down your leg all the way to the foot, numbness of weak muscles, and a general sense of feeling unwell.

If you have developed severe back pain for the first time and it is no better 10 days after onset, do not use this book or this chapter until you have consulted your doctor, physical therapist, or chiropractor.

INSTRUCTIONS

1. Immediately lie facedown.

If this is impossible because of pain intensity, go to bed. Attempt exercises next day.

2. When resting in bed, use a rolled towel or a night roll around your waist.

3. Perform McKenzie Method Exercises 1, 2, and 3. Every two hours, perform Exercises 1 and 2 once and Exercise 3 10 times. Perform Exercise 1 for two to three minutes, Exercise 2 for two to three minutes, and Exercise 3 10 times, which will take one to two minutes. (For details on all McKenzie back exercises, see Chapter 5.)

4. If the pain is more to one side and not decreasing: While lying facedown, move hips away from the painful side and do Exercises 2 and 3.

5. Rest as much as possible, correctly supported.

6. Do not bend forward for three to four days.

7. Sit perfectly at all times—use lumbar roll.

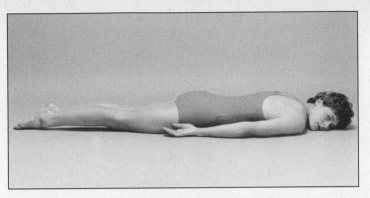

Figure P.1   Exercise 1

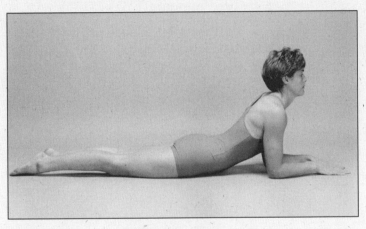

Figure P.2   Exercise 2

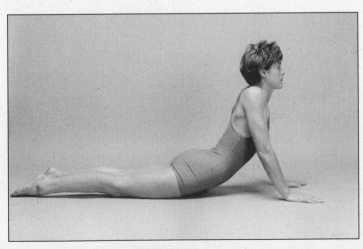

Figure P.3   Exercise 3

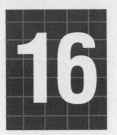

Panic Pages
for the Neck

In case of a sudden onset of acute neck pain, observe the following precautions. Then, if you can use this book, proceed with the instructions.

PRECAUTIONS

If you have developed neck pain for the first time and it is no better 10 days after onset, do not use this book or this chapter until you have consulted your doctor.

If you have complications to your neck problems, do not use this book or this chapter until you have consulted your doctor. Examples of complications are severe, stabbing pains, or that your head is pulled off-center, or that you have severe, continuing headaches.

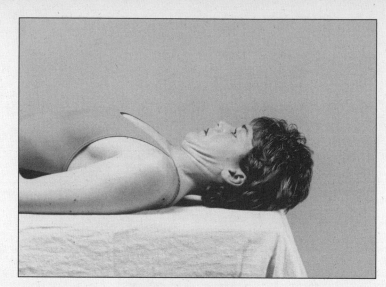

Figure P.4   *Exercise 3*

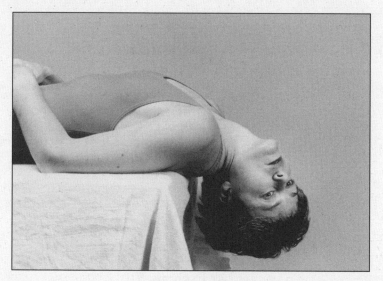

Figure P.5   *Exercise 4*

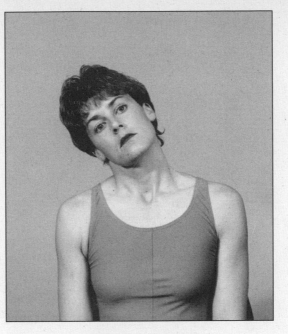

Figure P.6   *Exercise 5*

INSTRUCTIONS

1. Do not rest in bed. Keep your head as still as possible. Avoid all painful movements.
2. When sitting, use a lumbar roll to maintain a safe posture.
3. Do not bend the neck forward, roll the head around, or make quick movements of the head or neck.
4. First attempt Exercise 1. If Exercise 1 provides some relief, add Exercise 2. If, however, Exercise 1 has no effect or makes your symptoms worse, go immediately to Exercises 3 and 4, performing them every two hours. Do Exercise 3 10 times every two hours; do Exercise 4 once every two hours. (For details on all McKenzie neck exercises, see Chapter 12.)
5. When pain is more to one side and not responding to Neck Exercise 1, 2, 3, or 4, do Exercise 5, followed by Neck Exercises 1 and 2. Do Neck Exercises 5, 1, and 2 10 times every two hours.

Appendix A
How to Find a McKenzie-Trained Health Care Practitioner

To locate a physical therapist, chiropractor, or physician who is a credentialed member or associate of the McKenzie Institute International, telephone the Institute's U.S. branch at (800) 635-8380 or its Canadian branch at (800) 463-8568. You may also visit the McKenzie Institute's website at mckenziemdt.org.

Members of the McKenzie Institute worldwide are available to appear at schools to provide group education and instruction to schoolchildren in the correction of posture. The Institute has an educational video to assist in this program. There is no charge for either an appearance by a member of the Institute or the video. For further information, contact a credentialed member or associate of the McKenzie Institute.

The McKenzie Institute International Spinal Therapy and Rehabilitation Centers have been established for the purposes of providing treatment programs for patients with chronic and recurring back and neck problems.

There are now 21 McKenzie Institute branches serving 23 countries: Australia, Belgium, Brazil, Canada, Denmark, Finland, France, Germany, Greece/Cyprus, Hungary, Italy, Luxembourg, New Zealand, Nigeria, Poland, Russia, Sweden, Switzerland/Austria, the Netherlands, the United Kingdom, and the United States. Each branch includes faculty members who teach the McKenzie Method to practitioners.

The McKenzie Institute holds international conferences every two years. The most recent have been held in Cambridge, England, in August 1995;

Philadelphia in August 1997; and Maastricht, the Netherlands, in August 1999. In the intervening years, the U.S. branch holds a conference for North America. The most recent have been held in La Jolla (San Diego) in September 1996, New Orleans in August 1998, and Orlando in June 2000. At each international and North American conference, hundreds of doctors, physical therapists, and chiropractors gather to learn more about the McKenzie Method. There they also learn of the most current scientific literature as it pertains to conservative management of neck and lower back pain.

The McKenzie Institute provides two types of certification for health professionals already licensed by their states, provinces, or nations as physical therapists, chiropractors, or physicians. These are the Credentialing Certificate and the Credentialing Diploma. The certificate entitles the holder to use the term "Cert. M.D.T." (Certificate in Mechanical Diagnosis and Therapy) after his or her name; the diploma permits the use of "Dip. M.D.T." (Diploma in Mechanical Diagnosis and Therapy).

Requirements for the Certificate include a four-part series of courses and a written and practical examination that tests competency in diagnosis and treatment. Standards for the diploma are receipt of the certificate, completion of an 11-week residency program, and an advanced written and practical examination. In the United States alone, there are 472 health professionals holding the certificate or both the certificate and the diploma. States with large numbers of such health professionals include New York with 67, California with 38, Texas with 36, Pennsylvania with 32, New Jersey with 28, and Washington with 22.

Each year more than 60 McKenzie faculty in more than 25 countries train thousands of additional physical therapists and other practitioners in the McKenzie Method. Annually in the U.S. alone, 12 faculty members representing the McKenzie Institute train 2,300 practitioners. They do so in more than 120 courses in 35 cities. Worldwide, McKenzie Institute faculty have trained more than 20,000 physical therapists, chiropractors, and physicians.

The Institute works directly with referring physicians in formulating ongoing self-treatment programs tailored to the needs of specific individuals.

Further information about the Institute's programs is available at the telephone numbers and website noted at the beginning of this appendix.

Appendix B
Products for the Back and Neck

Sales of lumbar and cervical supports have generated substantial funding for education and research on back and neck pain. Grants have been made in countries including the United States, England, and Australia.

PRODUCTS FOR THE BACK

The value of a lumbar roll is discussed in Chapter 4 of this book. The Original McKenzie® Lumbar Roll is constructed of high-quality foam with a durable, gray, cotton/polyester cover and is available in two densities: Regular and Firm.

The newest version of the Original McKenzie® Lumbar Roll is the Original McKenzie® SuperRoll™, which provides long-life lumbar support without significant bulk. You can position the SuperRoll exactly where it is needed, and can secure it in place with either a hook-and-loop panel or a removable adjusting strap. This product is designed especially for automobiles and office chairs.

A wraparound lumbar roll for use when sleeping is also available: The Original McKenzie® Night Roll ties around the waist, presenting an ideal way to help correct sleeping position as described in Chapter 4 of this book. It is available in three sizes.

PRODUCT FOR THE NECK

Described in Chapter 10 of this book, The Original McKenzie® Cervical Roll supports the neck while you sleep. Designed to slip between your pillow and pillowcase, the cervical roll reduces strain on the cervical discs while providing greater comfort than is available from any pillow alone.

ORDERING INFORMATION

All of the rolls described in this book are available in North America only from Orthopedic Physical Therapy Products (OPTP) in Minneapolis, Minnesota, USA. For information, including pricing, you may call (612) 553-0452 or may write to OPTP; P.O Box 47009; Minneapolis, MN 55447-0009, USA. Orders may be placed by calling (800) 367-7393.

About the Author and the Collaborator

ROBIN McKENZIE

Without embellishment, Robin McKenzie can be called the most prominent physical therapist in the world, the one star in his field. Worldwide, more than 20,000 health professionals have been trained in McKenzie's methods. Authors praise him. International celebrities who have been treated by McKenzie-trained physical therapists do the same. Many Toyota Motor Corporation vehicles in New Zealand now use seats that McKenzie helped design.

A recent survey of 293 physical therapists completed by researchers at the University of Washington in Seattle concluded that the majority believe Robin McKenzie's approach is the single most useful way to treat back pain.

McKenzie is so well regarded in the medical, physical therapy, and chiropractic professions that there are now 21 McKenzie Institute International branches serving 23 countries: Australia, Belgium, Brazil, Canada, Denmark, Finland, France, Germany, Greece/Cyprus, Hungary, Italy, Luxembourg, New Zealand, Nigeria, Poland, Russia, Sweden, Switzerland/Austria, the Netherlands, the United Kingdom, and the United States. Each branch includes faculty members who teach the McKenzie Method to practitioners.

The McKenzie Institute holds international conferences every two years. The most recent have been held in Cambridge, England, in August 1995; Philadelphia in August 1997; and Maastricht, the Netherlands, in August 1999. In the intervening years, the U.S. branch holds a conference for North America. The most recent have been held in La Jolla (San Diego) in September 1996, New Orleans in August 1998, and Orlando in June 2000. At each international and North American conference, hundreds of doctors, physical therapists, and chiropractors gather to learn more about the McKenzie Method. There they also learn of the most current scientific literature as it pertains to conservative management of neck and lower back pain.

The McKenzie Institute provides two types of certification for health professionals already licensed by their states, provinces, or nations as physical therapists, chiropractors, or physicians. These are the Credentialing Certificate and the Institute Diploma in Mechanical Diagnosis and Therapy. The certificate entitles the holder to use the term "Cert. M.D.T." (Certificate in Mechanical Diagnosis and Therapy) after his or her name; the diploma permits the use of "Dip. M.D.T." (Diploma in Mechanical Diagnosis and Therapy).

Requirements for the certificate include a four-part series of courses and a written and practical examination that tests competency in diagnosis and treatment. Standards for the diploma are receipt of the certificate, completion of an 11-week residency program, and an advanced written and practical examination. In the United States alone, there are 472 health professionals holding the certificate or both the certificate and the diploma. States with large numbers of such health professionals include New York with 67, California with 38, Texas with 36, Pennsylvania with 32, New Jersey with 28, and Washington with 22.

Each year more than 60 McKenzie faculty in more than 25 countries train thousands of additional physical therapists and other practitioners in the McKenzie Method. Annually in the U.S. alone, 12 faculty members representing the McKenzie Institute train 2,300 practitioners. They do so in more than 120 courses in 35 cities. Worldwide, McKenzie Institute faculty have trained more than 20,000 physical therapists, chiropractors, and physicians.

Robin McKenzie has earned honors that set him apart from any other physical therapist in the world.

- In 1982 McKenzie was made an Honorary Life Member of the American Physical Therapy Association "in recognition of distinguished and meritorious service to the art and science of physical therapy and to the welfare of mankind." This association presents only about two honorary life memberships per year.

- In 1983 he was elected a member of the International Society for the Study of the Lumbar Spine. At the time, the society's membership was restricted to 150 members worldwide.

- In 1984 he was elected a Fellow of the American Back Society.

- In 1985 he was awarded an Honorary Fellowship by the New Zealand Society of Physiotherapists (physical therapists).

- In 1987 he was made an Honorary Life Member of the New Zealand Manipulative Therapists Association.

- In 1990 he became an Honorary Fellow of the Chartered Society of Physiotherapists of the United Kingdom.

- In 1990, in the Queen's Birthday Honours, Queen Elizabeth conferred on McKenzie the title Officer of the Most Excellent Order of the British Empire, entitling him to be addressed as "Robin McKenzie, O.B.E."

- In 1998, he became an Honorary Fellow of the New Zealand College of Physiotherapy.

- In 2000, in the New Year Honors, the Queen appointed him to an even higher order, naming him a Companion of the New Zealand Order of Merit (CNZM).

McKenzie has written two books for health professionals to use with patients being treated for back or neck pain, *Treat Your Own Back* and *Treat Your Own Neck*. The books are part of the treatment program for the patients. *Treat Your Own Back* has sold more than 3.5 million copies worldwide. *Treat Your Own Neck* has sold more than 2 million. McKenzie also has written three books for health professionals themselves: *The Lumbar Spine: Mechanical Diagnosis and Therapy*, *The Cervical Spine: Mechanical Diagnosis and Therapy*, and *The Human Extremities: Mechanical Diagnosis and Therapy*.

Among those who praise McKenzie are authors of other books on back and neck pain. Judylaine Fine is the founder of the Back Association of Canada, the only charitable foundation in North America devoted to educating back sufferers and those who treat them. She is the author of *Your Guide to Coping with Back Pain*. In that book she writes:

> The McKenzie Method approaches disc problems in a totally new way that focuses on soft tissue (mostly muscles and ligaments). . . . But its most revolutionary aspect is the use of extension exercises and the maintenance of the lumbar lordotic curve. . . .
>
> . . . [A]lmost everyone agrees that, for disc problems in particular, extension exercises should be part of the treatment. The fact that our current definition of good posture is dramatically different from what it was just a decade ago has a lot to do with Robin McKenzie.
>
> In 1983, Robin McKenzie became the first physical therapist to be elected to the membership of the prestigious Society for the Study of the Lumbar Spine. To many people, myself included, it felt as if the entire profession was being knighted, not just the man himself. . . . Physical therapists would never use the term, but I can say it: Robin McKenzie was the profession's first star.

COLLABORATOR

A former public interest attorney who switched careers to writing, Craig Kubey has published seven books, three of them national bestsellers (on *The New York Times* or other major lists). Reviewers have called two of Kubey's books the best ever published on their subjects. Among Kubey's books are *Pat Summerall's Sports in America* (HarperCollins, a book on 32 sports legends, a collaboration with sportscaster Pat Summerall), *You Don't Always Need a Lawyer* (Consumer Reports Books, a book on alternatives to lawsuits), *The Viet Vet Survival Guide* (Ballantine Books, a book instructing American military veterans on how to get government benefits, even if the government has unfairly denied their claims), and *The Winners' Book of Video Games* (Warner Books, a book on game strategy and the industry).

Kubey has benefitted dramatically from McKenzie's exercises for both the back and the neck.

Index

Page numbers in *italics* refer to exercise instructions